PERSONAL BEST

PERSONAL BEST

Train Your Brain
and
Transform Your Body for Life

Gloria Schwartz

The material in this book is for informational purposes only and is not intended as a substitute for the advice and care of your physician. It is intended to provide helpful and informative material on the subjects addressed in the publication. It is sold with the understanding that the author and publisher are not engaged in rendering medical, health, nutritional, or any other kind of personal professional services in this book. The reader should consult his or her medical, health, or other competent professional before adopting any of the suggestions in this book or drawing inferences from it. The author and the publisher expressly disclaim responsibility for any adverse effects that may result from the use or application of any of the information contained in this book.

Some names and identifying details have been changed to protect the privacy of individuals.

FIRST EDITION

Author's photo by Allan Wolfsohn

ISBN: 0992041104
ISBN-13: 978-0-9920411-0-6

Printed in the U.S.A.

DEDICATION

For my husband Allan and our sons Jesse and Joshua

If you will it, it is no dream.
—Theodor Herzl

CONTENTS

ACKNOWLEDGMENTS

I'd like to thank my husband, Allan Wolfsohn, for loving me through thick and thin, chauffeuring me to races, and waiting for me at every finish line.

Thanks to my sons Jesse and Joshua. They are my greatest treasures and the two most important reasons for taking care of myself.

Thank you to my sister-in-law Sima Goel for encouraging me to take charge of my health.

Special thanks to Peg McGowan for her copyediting skills, generosity, and enthusiasm.

Special thanks to Carol-Ann Savick for her attention to detail and the time and effort she generously contributed during the final review phase.

Thank you to the many people I've crossed paths with during my incredible journey and who have, in one way or another, encouraged or inspired me. Some of them are dear friends and others were only in my life for a moment in time, yet they each made an indelible mark and I am forever grateful.

PART I

7-POINT PLAN FOR SUCCESS

1 BLUEPRINT

Only you can decide if you will be successful.

I guess you could call it an epiphany. It just came to me. I realized at the age of 43 that I was out of shape, both physically and mentally. After gaining a few pounds year after year following the birth of my second son, I was no longer able to convince myself that I just had a little post-partum weight to lose; after all, my son was seven years old. The extra weight that I'd accumulated was the result of a sedentary lifestyle coupled with a lack of caring; at least, not caring about myself as much as I did before I had children. By not caring, I mean not making time for myself. I was spending 40 hours a week at a desk job in the high-pressure world of high tech. I was regularly taking extra work home to do after I tucked my boys Jesse and Joshua in for the night. Most spare time was primarily devoted to my family, including watching my sons play soccer while I cheered them on from the sidelines, watching them learn how to skate while I sat on a bench sipping hot chocolate, and watching them learn to swim while I sat on a chair and chatted with other parents. Note the pattern of sitting as my main activity.

I spent any remaining free time—and there wasn't much of it—exhausted in a semi-comatose, supine position on the couch, clutching the remote control in one hand and cookies or chips in the other. Cookies and chips were like non-judgmental friends. Cookies never told me I looked heavy. Chips never coaxed me to get up and move. I knew I was out of shape, tired and stressed, but I was not in a state of mental readiness to do anything serious about it.

1

Sure, the odd time I'd go to the gym to work out. That was usually in the evening, after a full day of work. I'd rush home to have supper with my husband Allan and our boys, and then drive to the gym. I was tired before I got there. I'd spend about 30 minutes walking on the treadmill. I'd half-heartedly use a few exercise machines. I didn't have goals or plans. I didn't have a workout program. I thought that by simply showing up at the gym, I was doing something good. On the way home, I'd pick up a little snack at the food court or the drive-thru—self-defeating but irresistible. I fooled myself into believing that if I didn't have fries with the hotdog or burger, then it was not that bad. I'd burn about 100 calories exercising and then I'd eat 500 or more calories on the way home. No wonder I wasn't seeing results. Of course, that made me feel like exercise was futile and I'd stop going to the gym for a few months.

This was a vicious cycle that went on for several years—a short spurt of misguided effort, followed by disappointment and a sense of failure. One time, I considered hiring a personal trainer to set me up with a program and coach me.

"Don't waste your money on a trainer. I can tell you for free that you look fat," quipped my colleague.

I thought about the cost of a training session. I thought about how many fast-food lunches I could get for that money. I didn't consider all of the benefits of having a trainer, probably because I was unaware of them. Because of my short-sightedness, I didn't hire a trainer and I didn't get the kind of direction, moral support, or physical results that would have kept me motivated.

My story is not unique; if you're reading this book, you've probably been through similar ups and downs.

❦

Today, I am 25 pounds lighter. My body composition has changed significantly. I'm more muscular and have less body fat. Because I increased my lean muscle mass, meaning I gained some muscle weight, I actually lost more than 25 pounds of fat. I'm six dress sizes smaller. I'm stronger. I'm more active. I feel more energetic. I'm more confident about my appearance. I'm enthusiastic about exercise. I feel happier and less stressed. I've pretty much conquered my addiction to junk food and I eat considerably healthier on a regular basis. I've adopted a holistic fitness lifestyle that encompasses a wide variety of physical activities and also addresses my emotional health and spiritual needs. I'm now a certified personal fitness trainer. I enjoy inspiring others through one-on-one training, group fitness instruction, public speaking, and writing.

What got me to change? What got me going? How did I cross the chasm from desk jockey, couch potato, and veritable fitness worrier to intrinsically-motivated fitness warrior?

Did I just wake up one day and decide that I love to exercise and no longer crave junk food? No! It's hard to change established patterns of behavior. My change process took about a year from the time I decided I had to do something, until I came to the point where I embraced exercise and adopted better eating habits as part of a lifestyle overhaul. My change process evolved into a journey of self-discovery and empowerment that has enriched my life. I learned how to train my brain and transform my body for life. My mission now is to help other people do the same—people just like you.

The purpose of this book is to share my story and help you embark on your own journey. I'll show you how to leverage valuable lessons from my experiences, including what worked well and mistakes I've made along the way. Throughout the book, I'll provide guidelines, tools, and best practices to help you succeed.

Many people can relate to me and to my experiences because I am "ordinary." Unlike the majority of fitness authors, I'm not an elite athlete or a record holder. I'm not a supermodel with an unrealistic, unattainable, digitally-enhanced body that symbolizes false perfection. My intention has never been to live a fringe or extremist lifestyle, to deprive myself of all of the pleasures associated with eating, to become the skinny woman that the media tries to make us believe is normal, or to have the androgynous shape of a prepubescent girl. I don't have an extremely muscular body like female models in muscle magazines. That's not an aesthetic I want for myself. I've never taken steroids or any other substance to increase my muscle definition.

I'm not at the other end of the spectrum either. My story doesn't involve losing hundreds of pounds. I was never obese. I haven't had any type of surgery to help me lose weight or to improve my appearance. No lifting, enlarging, snipping, or tucking. No liposuction. To each his own, but other than my hair color, I am all natural. What you see is the real me.

Unlike some people who work in the fitness industry, I don't hawk phoney or questionable products to make a quick buck, such as appetite suppressants, fat-burning pills, meal-replacement shakes, prepackaged meals, fad diets, or exercise gadgets. Unlike many popular self-help books of the same genre, my book title doesn't contain "quick," "easy," "10 minutes," "10 days," or similar marketing buzzwords to suggest that the journey you're about to embark on will be anything short of a challenge. I don't make false or exaggerated claims. I don't use gimmicks. I'll tell you right now that there are no quick fixes or shortcuts. Don't trust anyone who tries to convince you otherwise. There is no such thing as a one-size-fits-all solution. Everything I describe about my journey and what you can expect for yourself comes from a place of honesty and integrity.

Who am I then? I am everyone and anyone who has struggled. I am your friend, your sister, your co-worker. I am you. I am the person I used to be, only better than I once was. Each day, I continue to evolve.

Someone recently said to me, "Gloria, you were never *that* heavy. You were never *my* size." This woman was implying that it was easy for me to lose weight and get in shape. That assumption is wrong. I have had my share of struggles, some of them extremely difficult. The difference between that woman and me is that I figured out how to rise up and overcome my challenges. What is perhaps most compelling about my story is that I transformed myself on the inside and the outside. I underwent a metamorphosis of mind, body, and spirit. When the new me emerged, I also discovered my new purpose—to help you achieve your personal best!

The lifestyle you decide to adopt is a very personal choice. It's one that I cannot make for you, but I'm here to inspire you and to awaken you to the possibilities. I'm here to spread my message: if you focus on fitness and inner health, you can achieve your goals. I'm here to teach you how to be strong and drop the excuses. I'm also here to remind you to give yourself recognition for all the achievements, big and small, that you make on your journey.

I got fit. So can you! There's no magic pill. This book offers prescriptions and encouragement for common sense and hard work.

I've assembled practical, no-nonsense information that I gleaned from my own experiences, from research, and from working with clients who are on their own individual journeys.

I've thrown in a dose of humor because I think it should be fun to work on improving yourself. Of course, humor is, at times, a defence mechanism, a mask behind which pain, shame, or guilt sometimes hides—like going to the gym feeling out of place and out of shape, or suddenly realizing that you're stuck in a rut, you've given up hope, and you need help. Instead of crying, laugh. Finding the humor in tough situations can help you get through the dark times. Remember, laughing burns calories! So don't forget to laugh your head off, and maybe you'll laugh off some of your fat too.

I think it's essential that I speak the truth, even if that sometimes means a no-holds-barred attitude. Coddling is ineffective. Compassion coupled with a firm hand gets results. It took lots of hard work to get fat and it's going to take lots of hard work to get fit. It took years of overeating and inactivity to get into a deconditioned state. It will take time and effort to do damage control and begin to turn things around. You can't blame anyone but yourself. Only when I finally took ownership of my negative thoughts and behaviors was I able to turn my situation around. I know you can do it too.

My story provides valuable insights that have practical applications. If you read it with an open mind, you can overcome your inner struggles that are preventing you from getting fit.

Where do you want to go on your journey? Who do you want to become? When I began my journey, I wasn't sure what I wanted. I hoped something inside of me would click, so that I'd feel motivated enough to eat better and to exercise a few times per week. And I wanted, eventually, to look better and be healthier.

Over time, my expectations became clearer. I wanted to have a trim, lean figure with some muscle tone. I wanted upper arms that didn't keep flapping long after I'd stopped waving good-bye. I wanted a reasonably flat stomach that I didn't have to suck in when I zipped up my pants. I wanted to eat nutritious foods that were good for me, yet continue to enjoy some of the little pleasures in life like chocolate. I wanted a lifestyle that got me off the couch doing a variety of physical activities that I could actually enjoy. I wanted to be able to incorporate these activities into my life without feeling that I was suffering or bored. I wanted to be able to walk into a gym and feel like I belonged. I wanted to look in a full-length mirror and smile rather than cringe, even if I was trying on a bathing suit. I never wanted to be perfect, just better.

I now have all of the things that I wanted—and so much more! I've earned them. I'm better in many ways than I was a few years ago.

This book is my labor of love. It gives me great pleasure knowing that you're reading it. I believe it can change your life for the better. This book is a gift to myself on the occasion of my fiftieth birthday. My story is a celebration of what each of us can achieve at any stage of life when we live with courage and conviction. I am more fit now than I was 10, even 20 years ago. I have achieved my personal best. Looking forward, I know the best is yet to come.

If you're willing to apply what you learn from this book with genuine commitment to yourself, you too can achieve your personal best!

❦

Let's think of getting fit as a project. Having worked in project management for many years, I know that a good predictor of success is having a well-defined plan. Therefore, the first point of my practical 7-Point Plan for Success is, in fact, to have a plan to begin with! Just as an architect creates a beautiful structure by starting with a carefully crafted blueprint, so too, can you design your body. A blueprint is a framework in which you assemble pieces of a puzzle and watch the big picture become clearer.

One of the greatest artists of all time said, "I saw the angel in the marble and then I carved until I set him free." As Michelangelo chiseled away, the statue of *David* emerged. Michelangelo had a vision. His hard work, commitment, and passion brought out the best. As your thinking evolves, you'll believe more in yourself and your potential. It is then, like Michelangelo did with *David*, that you'll be able to work with passion to carve out your best self.

Because the body and the mind are intertwined, the blueprint that I propose takes a holistic approach rather than just addressing your physical issues. I must confess that I didn't have a blueprint when I began my journey. In retrospect, a blueprint from someone like me—someone I could relate to—someone who had travelled the road upon which I was about to embark, would have helped me tremendously. Instead, I went through a steep, time-consuming learning curve. I hit many bumps along the way. Initially, I cobbled together tips and ideas from numerous sources. Eventually, I constructed a framework out of a series of strategies for success, and I used my personal experiences as the glue. I want to share my blueprint with you because it will put you on the right track. I'll be honest—it won't *guarantee* success. Only you can decide if you will be successful. I can't do all of the work for you, but I can improve your odds of success.

As you construct your individual and unique blueprint, I'll teach you how to incorporate each of the following components:

- Becoming mentally prepared for change by understanding what stage of readiness you're currently in, and learning how to consciously progress to a more advanced stage.

- Setting effective short- and long-term goals, and learning how to identify and overcome obstacles.

- Gaining knowledge about food by understanding the difference between a diet and a lifestyle, understanding the underlying reasons for your problematic eating patterns, and learning how to make informed and mindful choices.

- Exploring different kinds of exercises and activities, and discovering what you enjoy and what helps keep you motivated to stay active.

- Cultivating an environment rich in role models, mentors, and emotional support.

- Developing maintenance skills that will enable you to stay focused and committed for your lifetime.

Gloria Schwartz

Personal Best Exercises

o   Are you willing to take ownership of your behaviors?

o   Are you ready to figure out what you really want?

o   Are you prepared to work hard and earn what you desire?

Did you know?

•   A blueprint consists of components, plans, and strategies. It encourages proactive, rather than reactive, behaviors.

•   A blueprint will help you navigate the confusing worlds of fitness and nutrition, and make better decisions.

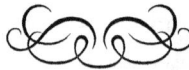

2 PREPAREDNESS

It is possible to use lifestyle as a tool to change your destiny.

Are you ready and willing to make a real commitment to yourself, to devote time and attention to yourself, and to learn how to eat better and exercise? Is your ultimate goal to optimize your health? Are you truly prepared to change your lifestyle and hence, your life? A blueprint and good intentions aren't enough. When you are mentally prepared for change, you can attain it *and* maintain it. You have to believe before you can achieve.

"Dream lofty dreams, and as you dream, so shall you become," wrote James Allen in his classic inspirational book *As a Man Thinketh*, originally published in 1902 (2008, p. 38).

Important processes require mental preparedness. I prefer the term *preparedness* rather than the more colloquial term *readiness* because preparedness is often used in reference to a state of readiness for war. The emotional and physical challenges ahead may feel like a battle, but victory awaits. Part of the change process is learning to unleash your inner warrior so you can overcome your fears and fight a good fight.

Learning how to ride a bike, trying a new food, or applying for a challenging job—these are examples of things we do in life that require us to be mentally prepared. Have you ever seen (or been) a parent trying to coax their child to jump into the deep end of the pool to no avail? Yet, one day, this same child suddenly decides to jump in on his own, not once, but repeatedly. The child was mentally prepared for that big moment—a moment of change that took him from standing fearfully at the edge of the pool to leaping into the water. I remember being that child and that parent. It's the same idea for moving forward with a plan for self-improvement. Sometimes knowledge—for example, knowing the basic facts about nutrition and the benefits of exercise—is not enough to persuade us to act. We need to be in a state of mind where we are ready to commit. We need a sense of urgency to take action.

How many times have you (and I) bought diet and recipe books, joined a gym, read magazine articles featuring miraculous weight-loss stories, bought a cartload of healthy food, made New Year's resolutions to lose weight or get active, or swore we'd stop buying fast-food lunches and start brown-bagging healthy ones? Why have so many of the promises that we made to ourselves gone unfulfilled? Because we were not ready! We had the facts. We knew what to do, or so we thought. We spent money to get the equipment and food and gym membership. So why didn't we follow through? If we did act, why were our actions short-lived? We were not mentally prepared to step out of our comfort zones, to acknowledge our shortcomings, and to change ourselves from within.

You can't buy fitness or health. I used to think that if I just had a personal trainer to whip me into shape and a personal chef to force me to eat healthy meals, I'd be perfect, and it would be so easy to be lean and fit. I've learned that money or other resources can't replace a state of mental readiness. You need to become intrinsically motivated. Experts definitely help, but it's up to you to do most of the work. You can't expect someone else to take care of your body and mind. Look at Oprah. She's one of the wealthiest women in the world. She has chefs, personal trainers, and just about every kind of assistant and coach imaginable. Yet, she goes through cycles of extreme weight loss and weight gain. Why is it so hard to maintain a healthy lifestyle?

Your success depends on your state of mental preparedness. That's one of the secrets I figured out.

According to the *Transtheoretical Model* of *Change* (James Prochaska and Carlo DiClemente, 1983), there are different stages of mental readiness for changing your health-related behavior:

- Pre-contemplation: If you are in the Pre-contemplation stage, lifestyle changes are not even on your radar. Perhaps you're just reading this book because you found it on a coffee table. More likely, if you were in this stage, you wouldn't have bothered to give this book more than a passing glance. People in this stage are unwilling or resistant to change. They are in denial or ignorant of their problems.

- Contemplation: If you're in the Contemplation stage, you're just starting to think about improvements like exercising or changing your dietary habits; however, you may be ambivalent and you haven't yet taken any steps towards making changes.

- Preparation: If you're in the Preparation stage, you've done more than think; you've taken some preparatory steps in the right direction. Perhaps you've toured a gym and asked about membership prices, or you've purchased a pair of running shoes.

- Action: Once you're in the Action stage, you're actively modifying your behavior or the environment to overcome your problems. You may have modified some of your eating habits. You may have started taking a fitness class or begun going for regular walks with a buddy.

- Maintenance: As time passes, usually six months or more, and such behaviors become habitual, you enter the Maintenance stage. The Maintenance stage is a psychologically fragile stage. It's common to have a relapse for a period of time that may be brief or last for years. Sometimes lack of motivation, change in schedule, a vacation, a new baby, an illness, financial problems, or other situations can interfere with this stage.

The authors of the Transtheoretical model later came up with a sixth and final stage that they referred to as the Termination stage. That's when you have no desire to return to your unhealthy lifestyle or habits, and you feel assured that you'll keep up a healthy lifestyle forever. Some researchers claim that this stage is rarely achieved. In my opinion, this stage implies perfection. I don't believe we can ever be perfect.

Relapsing at any stage is a distinct possibility. In fact, it's common. Despite feelings of disappointment when this occurs, a relapse is not a failure. I'm going to help you develop the necessary skills to get into the Maintenance stage. Essentially, I want to "convert" you. I want to empower you to maintain a healthy lifestyle —for life! I'm going to arm you with strategies that will help you deal with your day-to-day challenges. If you relapse, you'll be better equipped to return through the stages and back into Maintenance as quickly and seamlessly as possible.

What's the catalyst that will enable you to become mentally prepared and ready to follow a blueprint for success? There is no universal answer. For each person, the trigger may be different. What was my catalyst? What got me going? How did I transition from being inactive to running half marathons? Before I tell you, let me take a step back and explain what brought me to a place where I knew I had to make some serious changes.

Growing up, I was academically inclined. I loved school. I loved learning. My parents encouraged and supported me as I pursued a bachelor's degree in psychology, followed by a master's degree in educational technology. I then had a career for nearly 20 years in software training development.

As my career evolved, I advanced to a management position and took on more responsibilities. I was very satisfied with my position and duties. I discovered that along with this success came some negatives—longer hours at the office, taking extra work home, and increased pressures and stress. I wasn't just responsible for what I was working on; I was responsible for the work delivered by my team. I loved what I was doing, but there was a price to pay. I found myself eating more fast food for lunch, and making a beeline for the vending machine mid-afternoon for sugary and fatty snacks. I knew that I'd be healthier if I brought a homemade lunch to work and avoided the vending machine; but I became indifferent. I couldn't be bothered. The junk food was convenient and tasted good. How bad could it be? After all, I considered myself average weight when I looked around at my colleagues.

Because I'd been slim most of my life, when I started gaining a few pounds here and there in my late thirties, I continued to perceive myself as slim. The weight crept up slowly over several years, so I barely noticed the difference. Sure, the scale couldn't lie, nor did the size of my clothing, but I didn't feel "fat." I rationalized that it was not *that* bad to eat the way I was eating. It was not *that* bad to sit at a desk most of the day. I told myself that I didn't have time to exercise on my lunch break, yet somehow I regularly found time to go out for fast food. Occasionally, I'd fool myself by going for a walk at lunch with some coworkers, but we typically ended up at the donut shop where we'd have donuts or calorie-packed iced coffee drinks. Over the years, those extra calories added up. In retrospect, those daily indulgences were stress-induced, and akin to a junkie getting a fix.

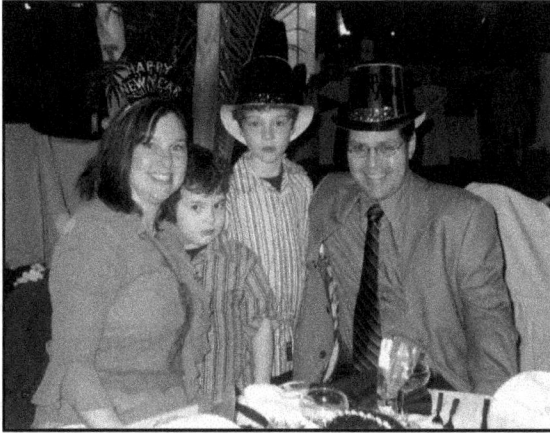

Celebrating my 42nd birthday with Joshua, Jesse, and Allan at the end of 2005. I wasn't yet ready to address my weight or health issues.

Out of the blue, in September 2006, I was laid off from my job, along with about 200 colleagues. I was stunned. Everything I had believed in was no longer true—hard work, commitment, consistently contributing to the company's bottom line—none of this suddenly mattered to senior management. For years, I'd been led to believe by my superiors that I was essential to the department. I knew no one is indispensable, but it became a painful realization that I was nothing more than a cog in a giant wheel when I was escorted out the door after 11 years of dedicated service.

I took the job loss hard. At first I was in shock. Then I became depressed. I had nightmares and I cried often. My ego and my sense of self had been intricately tied to my career. Even though I was a wife, a mother, a sister, a daughter, and a friend, I suddenly felt like I was a nobody.

Work had been a social outlet for me too. Many of my colleagues had become friends. What would I do at home alone, with my husband at work, my children at school, and my friends at work?

Nearly all of my friends had careers. That's what seemed normal to me. I never had the desire to be one of those women who, for whatever reason, didn't work outside the home. Now I was one of them.

I told myself that I mustn't let this reactive depression take hold of me. Two options immediately came to mind that first morning of unemployment: I could take up drinking and drown my sorrows, or I could get out of bed, get dressed, and go to the gym. Since I'm one shot short of a teetotaler, I decided that the best thing I could do was to force myself to start going to the gym, just to have a destination each morning. The gym was located in the community center right next to my sons' school. Now that I had all this free time, I could do some exercise—something to get myself out of the house and out of the blues.

You may think that I was blessed, given the luxury of all this unexpected freedom. I didn't see it that way for quite some time. I felt punished. My hard-earned position in a top high tech company had been unfairly ripped away from me.

My few non-working homemaker acquaintances told me I was lucky to get a break. One said that not working is the best-kept secret. Another said that working is overrated. I should take the time to do things for myself, they advised.

"Like what?" I asked. One woman suggested I use my time to clean out a closet. I could do that in an hour, but then what? I knew she meant well, but I was rather annoyed. Others suggested I take painting classes, read a good book, or volunteer to serve hotdogs at my sons' school lunches. I'd been so career-oriented. The tasks they suggested seemed frivolous and demeaning.

When I got laid off, I received a generous severance package. I was to receive full pay and benefits for 11 months—one month per year of service. If I were to take a new job elsewhere during this period, the remainder of the package would be cut off. So, as they say, it was the best of times, it was the worst of times. I was getting paid and not having to work for it, but I wanted to go back to work. I was not motivated to take a new job because I'd lose part of my package. I was truly torn. I didn't even know if I'd be marketable at the age of 42. I lost all self-confidence overnight, even though I'd been very self-assured and felt competent all those years in the workforce. I applied for management positions just to see what would happen. I landed several job offers surprisingly quickly. This was great for renewing my confidence.

Allan encouraged me to turn down the job offers, take a year off, and enjoy myself. I reluctantly decided to heed his advice and take the full financial package. I'd find something to do for that time, I told myself. But what? How fulfilling could a watercolor course be? What sense of accomplishment would I possibly get from walking on a treadmill or lifting some dumbbells?

"What do you do all day?" I queried several women at the gym. "Oh, I run here, I run there. I'm always busy," declared Sandy, the mother of two boys who were in the same grades as my sons. Run here? Run there? Where in the world was she running all day? The grocery store? The hair salon? The gym? How much of that can one do? How would I fill my days? How would I feel engaged and fulfilled? I'd always found work satisfying. That's all I'd ever known. I'm no Martha Stewart—baking cookies and cleaning toilets do not turn my crank. I could only do so much of that.

It would take time, but my tune would change. I wouldn't have believed it then, but I would eventually find myself in a state of mind where my days seemed too short; where I wanted to exercise and actually felt passionate about it; where I was in control of my eating (most of the time), rather than my eating habits in control of me; and where I was investing in myself and becoming a better me.

❧

So, what was the secret for me? What got me in a state of mental readiness to pursue an improved lifestyle? The secret for me was that I started caring. It didn't happen immediately; as a matter of fact, it took a long time. When I was a career person, I thought that improving myself meant getting my hair highlighted or a manicure— little feel-good perks. There's nothing wrong with that as long as you don't neglect your health. I didn't realize then what I've come to know—I must love myself enough to take care of more than just the superficial. I must take care of my whole self—mind, body, and spirit. No one else can do it for me.

Unfortunately, for the first year after I lost my job, I went to the gym sporadically, mainly as something to do to kill time. Isn't it sad when you have the luxury of time and you just want to kill it? Time can never be recovered. Yet, I was squandering it, until I came to a point where I made up my mind to view my freedom and luxury of time as an unexpected gift rather than as a punishment. That's when I finally got serious about fitness.

But there was more to it than that. There was another key ingredient that contributed to my success. When I started on what turned out to be an amazing journey, I acted, in part, out of fear. I have been asked many times what prompted me to modify my lifestyle. What was the trigger? I could never truly answer that question. It's not that I didn't know; it's that I wasn't ready to speak the truth. I didn't want pity, sympathy, or any other kind of negative attention.

Now that I'm fearless—and by that I don't mean completely devoid of fear, but rather able to address and overcome my fears—I can share the whole truth. It's something that only a few people know about me—until now.

When I was 31 years old, Allan and I applied for life insurance. That required us to undergo routine medical assessments. At that time, my urine test came back as abnormal. One thing led to another and I soon found myself visiting a nephrologist—a kidney specialist. I was diagnosed with a chronic form of kidney disease. I was shocked. I'd felt fine. I didn't have any symptoms. I was young. I was slim. I didn't have any risk factors such as diabetes or a family history of kidney disease. I'd never had a kidney infection or any serious illness. The doctor couldn't establish a cause.

I wondered then whether emotional distress could cause bodily damage such as kidney disease. I had been emotionally distraught since the death of my beloved mother from cancer the year before. Perhaps that psychological trauma had taken a physical toll and manifested itself in this way. Maybe I was born with a weakness in my kidneys or I was unknowingly exposed to some virus or toxic substance that, at some point, caused damage to the nephrons (the microscopic filters in the kidneys). Whatever the cause, the fact was that my kidneys were damaged and there was no way to repair them. Even worse, the nephrologist informed me that my kidney function would continue to decline over the years.

The nephrologist told me there was nothing I could do. She informed me that I would eventually require kidney replacement therapy—dialysis or a transplant. I was devastated. I didn't like that pessimistic prognosis, so I found a new nephrologist. At that time, Allan and I didn't yet have children. The new doctor encouraged me to start a family while my kidneys were still functioning relatively well. He said I would be followed closely at the high-risk pregnancy unit.

The new nephrologist put me on a daily blood pressure pill. He said that the only treatment to try to extend the life of my kidneys was to keep my blood pressure lower than normal. Reduced kidney function can contribute to high blood pressure and high blood pressure can further damage the kidneys—a vicious cycle.

The years went by. I had two healthy sons in my mid-thirties, Jesse and Joshua. Because of my medical situation, both pregnancies were complicated and both babies had to be delivered prematurely. I had to be induced both times because I was getting preeclampsia— elevated blood pressure that could be life-threatening to my unborn children and to me. In fact, my nephrologist had suggested I not have a second child as it was risky. Being stubborn by nature, I accepted the risk. I'm thankful it all worked out well.

Life went on and I tried not to dwell on my health problems, but I couldn't help it. It was a constant, underlying stressor. My nephrologist retired and a younger one took his place. He told me to watch my sodium and protein intake and to remain on the blood pressure medication, but that was it. He said there was nothing further he or I could do.

I felt that I didn't have enough guidance. I felt helpless. As a result, I gave up and ate pretty much whatever I wanted. Between my career and my family, I was busier than ever. My weight slowly began to creep up.

I continued to visit the nephrologist once or twice a year and had blood and urine tests, a kidney biopsy, and various other tests. Apart from these occasional appointments, there wasn't much to do. At least, that's what the medical professionals led me to believe. Doctors are trained to prescribe medication. I eventually came to understand that a healthy lifestyle can prevent, as well as slow the progression of, many diseases.

About one year after I was laid off from work, my doctor estimated that—based on the rate of decline in my kidney function— my kidneys would fail within five years. He suggested I talk to family and friends about my situation and start looking for a potential kidney donor. I'd just turned 44 years old.

I was more scared than when I was initially diagnosed years earlier, because I now had two young children to think of. Who would take care of them if I was incapacitated, if I had to be on dialysis three times per week indefinitely, or, if I was lucky enough to get a kidney donor and had to be hospitalized? Even worse, what if I died from complications? My head was spinning and overflowing with negative thoughts. I was in tears.

I broke the bad news to Allan. Unlike me, he's an optimist. He comforted me and advised me not to worry or panic. But how could I not worry?

The next time I was in Montreal, I visited my sister-in-law Sima. I broke down crying as I told her what the nephrologist had said. She insisted that I not believe him. She said that his words were not the words of God. She had a lot more to say. Sima is a chiropractor and wellness professional. She advised me to take better care of myself and take charge of my life, to enjoy life, and not to worry so much. At that time, I knew she meant well, but I felt it was easy for her to be positive. She was healthy. I was not. I felt as though there was a black cloud over my head.

While I didn't initially agree with everything Sima had to say, I did agree that I should take better care of myself. I made up my mind to get into better shape. I rationalized that when my kidneys eventually failed, at least the rest of me would be in better health and I'd be more likely to overcome the medical hurdles that I would face. I decided that if I was going to go down, I'd go down fighting!

My doctor never prescribed exercise or healthy eating. Yes, he suggested I lose a few pounds and watch my protein and sodium intake, but even the nephrology dietician that I met with from time to time told me I could continue eating fast food and drinking cola. He just advised me to have those things a little less often. Neither of them gave me tough love. They never said, "Gloria, get your act together. Heal yourself. Don't act helpless and hopeless. Don't eat crap every day because you've given up. And stop imagining the worst." Sima had the sense and the courage to talk to me like that.

Still, it took me a long time, several pep talks, and lots of self-help books to realize that I'd been wasting precious time—years, actually—worrying about what might happen, when I should be enjoying my health and blessed life in the present.

Sima encouraged me to get started, to continue exercising but also to watch what I was eating. She persisted until I became receptive to the idea of change. And so I slowly started with a few baby steps, a few small changes. I didn't realize that I was embarking on a journey of training my brain and transforming my body for life.

⚜

As each month passed, I mentally counted down from the five years that the nephrologist had projected my kidneys would last. I kept thinking about that five-year mark and scratching off months in my mind, fearing that dreaded deadline. I felt like time was running out. I wanted to travel more while I was physically well enough to do so. I felt like I couldn't make big plans because of the terrible deadline that was looming. I believed that kidney failure in five years was inevitable. I ruminated about worst-case scenarios even though I had worked for many years with a man who had a successful kidney transplant and was enjoying a full life.

I didn't go back to work—even after my severance package ran out—because I wanted to spend as much time as possible with my children while I felt well. I enjoyed life and smiled on the outside, but on the inside I was scared and anxious about the future. Ironically, during that period, I felt physically better than ever because I got myself into the best shape of my life and I was motivated to step outside of my comfort zone.

About two years after I truly committed to a fit lifestyle and had achieved many goals, I had one of my routine appointments with my doctor. I was terrified that he'd announce that my kidney function had declined even more and that I would soon need dialysis. On that dreaded day in February 2010, the doctor came into the room with a big grin on his face.

"Everything is stable. You've defied all odds," he announced. He said that the various indicators had not gotten any worse in the last couple of years. "Whatever you are doing, keep it up." I was shocked. When I saw him a couple of years prior, he had told me that my kidneys would likely fail in five years. Now he was singing a different tune. I felt like a black cloud was lifted off of my shoulders. I then showed the dietician a record of everything I had eaten in a month and he was quite pleased. I had given up fast food and pop and was focused on making my body healthier.

When I phoned Sima to share my good news, she suggested that I share it with the world. I should use this experience to show others who may be in a similar situation—suffering from a health issue or living with a challenge that they feel is outside of their control—that it is possible to use lifestyle as a tool to improve one's life, even change one's destiny! She said I should spread a message of hope and empowerment. She believed that my new lifestyle had positively impacted my disease. The impossible had become possible, or, as she says, "Miracles can happen."

Had I charted a new course for myself? I can't say for sure whether it was my lifestyle, luck, or divine intervention that contributed to the change in pattern of my kidney function over the past few years; but in 2013—five years after the start of my new lifestyle—that same nephrologist showed me more encouraging test results. All of those years when I neglected my health, my kidney function declined considerably. Once I began to take charge of my body, the progression of the disease slowed and then seemed to plateau.

Certainly, losing excess weight had reduced the strain on my kidneys. Getting fit had been good for my entire body, such as my blood pressure. My doctor even reduced the dosage of my blood pressure medication. Improving my diet had been good for my cholesterol levels and frankly, all of me. Being active and fit and challenging myself physically was reducing stress. Stress hormones are damaging to the body. As I saw health improvements, my attitude changed from negative to positive. I was no longer living in a gray world. I was no longer living in fear. My mind and body were in happy mode. My body was thanking me and rewarding me. I was receiving the gifts of better health and joy. I had worked hard for them. With those test results, I felt like I was born again.

To reiterate, my secret for success was to care about myself, to make *me* a priority. The enlightening realization that I must love and honor myself became my catalyst for meaningful and lasting change. Once the ball got rolling, there was no stopping me.

Personal Best Exercises

o   Identify the stage of readiness for change that you're in now.

o   Do you truly care about yourself and believe you deserve optimal health and wellness?

o   Are you willing to make yourself a priority?

Did you know?

•   Any author or product claiming you can lose weight or get fit without having to adhere to a balanced diet and regular exercise is more interested in profiting off of you than helping you.

•   Change often requires a gradual progression of small steps.

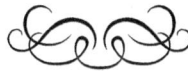

3 GOALS

When you're truly committed to achieving your goals, nothing will stop you.

A major component of the blueprint is goal setting. In order to achieve goals, you have to first establish them. The best way to start is to think of some short-term and long-term goals. Short-term goals are ones that you can accomplish in approximately three to six months; long-term goals in six to twelve months.

When thinking about goals, be realistic. You risk setting yourself up for failure if you expect to change every aspect of your diet, or if you try to change overnight from being inactive to running a marathon. In time, incremental changes to your lifestyle can have a transformational impact on your health, fitness, and appearance. As you achieve and build upon each short-term goal, your long-term goals will become more realistic.

You can even set a stretch goal—an extremely difficult goal you can only dream of right now because you don't know how to reach it. A stretch goal requires much more than just working hard. It is unachievable simply by doing what you already do but better. A stretch goal requires extending yourself to the limit and thinking and behaving in new and creative ways.

Once you have some goals in mind, document them. By writing them down, you clarify them. More importantly, you make a psychological commitment on paper (or electronically). You can see in words what you want to achieve. You can make revisions over time as needed.

Declaring your goals to other people has been shown to be an effective motivator. Tell your family or some friends about your goals. Don't keep them a secret. Don't let fear of failure hold you back from sharing your goals. I can tell you from experience that once I had the courage to declare my goals, I suddenly felt truly committed to them. It's almost like there's no going back.

Consider the reason behind each of your goals. Ask yourself why you want to achieve this or that. For a weight-loss goal, do you want to fit into your bathing suit on your upcoming vacation? Or do you want to lose weight to improve your health and make daily activities easier to perform? We all want to look good, but when appearance is the primary reason behind a goal, motivation may not be long-lasting. What will happen when you get back from your beach vacation? Will you still be dedicated to your weight-loss goal then?

By investing some time upfront to plan for your success, you'll increase your confidence and feel more engaged; those effects, in turn, will increase your odds of success.

When I decided to write my first set of goals, I sat down at my computer, put my fingers on the keyboard, and realized I didn't know what my goals were. I started thinking about what I would like to accomplish. Some of the goals I came up with pertained to physical and intellectual self-improvement. For example, I decided to set a goal of running a half marathon (21.1 kilometers). This was a distance I could never have imagined a year before when I was sedentary and could barely run one block without gasping for air. It would have seemed impossible. Now that I was more fit and could already run five to eight kilometers, it seemed like a stretch goal that would require serious training, dedication, and mental fortitude. Yet, it seemed within reach. I didn't know anything about races so I looked online to find out when a half marathon would take place in my city. It was early summer, and one was coming up in September, so I put that down as my target.

Within about an hour of starting to think of goals, I also came up with a goal to read more self-help books. I had read several over the preceding few months. One book that made a big impression on me and helped change my way of thinking for the better was *The Monk Who Sold His Ferrari* (1997). Some of the lessons I gleaned from that book were that I must figure out who and what really matter to me and I should spend more time with those people and on those activities. I also learned that to get anywhere, you have to overcome your fear and live life fully. That book gave me permission to focus on myself and devote time to strength training and running without feeling guilty. I also took away that I should devote more time to something I've always enjoyed—writing. That lesson was part of the decision-making process that led to authoring this book.

What kinds of goals should you start with? That's a very personal decision. Lots of people have a goal in mind. When I ask clients to tell me one of their goals off the top of their head, they often state things like "Lose 50 pounds." This sample statement has several flaws. First, it's vague. It doesn't indicate a target deadline, or an action plan. It's also a big goal. It's better to have realistic interim goals that lead up to a bigger, long-term goal.

When I work on goal-setting with clients, I help them set achievable ones using the SMART acronym. SMART is commonly used for defining goals. SMART stands for Specific, Measurable, Attainable, Realistic, and Time-bound goals.

An example of a vague goal is, "I'll walk for exercise." A SMART version of this goal might be, "Within three months, I'll be able to walk four kilometers non-stop in 30 minutes or less." With a SMART goal, you have a timeframe and other measures you can use to assess if you have achieved your goal.

Once you have a goal, you need a plan. In this example, perhaps you set aside some time four to five times per week to go for a walk. At first you might start with just 10 minutes if you're out of shape, then build up your endurance and speed slowly and safely over time.

Here is an extract from the first set of goals I wrote for myself in June of 2008:

- Run from the cottage to the mailbox (8 kilometers round trip) on extremely hilly dirt roads. Criteria: Complete without stopping. Target completion date: End of August.

- Lose five pounds by cutting back on junk food and by exercising six days per week. Criteria: Get down to 135 pounds. Target completion date: End of September.

- Do one proper chin-up. (This may not sound like much but it's a very demanding exercise, especially for women). Criteria: With fully extended arms, pull all the way up until chin is over the bar. Target completion date: End of December.

- Run a half marathon. Criteria: Complete it. Race time is irrelevant. Target completion date: End of September.

As the weeks and months passed, I referred to my goals periodically, adding information about my progress. I made a plan for each goal. When I accomplished a goal, I checked it off and set a new one. For example, for the half marathon goal, I added the following updates:

- As of August 5, I can run 12 kilometers in 90 minutes.

- As of September 2, I can run 19 kilometers in 2 hours and 25 minutes.

- On September 21, I ran the half marathon in 2 hours and 33 minutes. Goal accomplished!

Each goal required hard work and focus. To lose five pounds, I had to be more mindful of what kind of food I was eating. My plan for that goal included a commitment to reducing my restaurant visits to once a week. I didn't banish all processed food from my home. Instead, I took baby steps. I stopped eating in fast-food restaurants cold turkey. I found this very tough at first. I managed to get through the withdrawal symptoms such as cravings and agitation. I employed self-discipline by driving by, rather than through, the drive-thru. Eventually I lost interest in greasy burgers and fries and I felt more comfortable with some of my new eating habits. I then set some new goals, such as limiting the poor quality snacks I was consuming, and replacing them with better choices such as fresh veggies and fruit.

Incremental goals are those that we can better visualize and achieve. This allows us to travel a path of small successes that build upon one another, rather than bite off a huge challenge that we can't realistically attain in one shot.

Once you establish some preliminary goals, how do you measure your successes and failures? For example, if I hadn't bothered to exercise for a few days, or if I fell off the wagon and scoffed down a family-size bag of chips, was I a failure? Did I throw in the towel? Absolutely not!

We can learn from our failures—or as I prefer to call them, our mistakes and disappointments—and deposit what we learn into our knowledge bank. If you deem yourself a failure every time you're disappointed, you'll never accomplish anything. Accept minor setbacks, consider them lessons learned, and move on.

What are some things that we can measure, things that would easily let us know if we are succeeding? The obvious one is weight. I recommend that you start your program by having a trainer or a trusted friend measure your neck, chest/bust, waist at the smallest part, hips, upper arms, thighs, and calves. Write down those numbers, as well as your weight. If you're embarrassed, get over it! You won't be able to track your progress without benchmarks.

When I eventually hired a personal trainer, one of the first things I asked her was to take my measurements. Gina told me that most of her clients don't want to know their measurements. I wasn't embarrassed to let her measure me even though she looked like a blond Barbie with legs longer than my list of dietary no-nos. I was there for a reason—to get in shape. Before you can improve yourself, you need to admit the problem, and being overweight is reflected by your measurements. I eagerly wrote down the numbers as my starting point and tucked the slip of paper away for future reference. If you have the courage to do the same, you can have your measurements taken again in a few months and compare the numbers to what you first wrote down. When you start to see results by comparing the numbers, you'll be glad you recorded them.

The number on your bathroom scale reflects your total body weight, not your body composition. Your weight includes your muscle, fat, bones, water, and organs. When you regularly engage in strength-training exercises, you gain muscle mass. That's a good thing! So don't focus solely on your weight. If you stick to a healthy eating plan and continue with regular exercise, you'll improve your body composition—less fat and more muscle.

I noticed I went through times when my weight came to a plateau for a few weeks. When this happened, I modified my exercises, either by increasing the duration, frequency, or level of intensity, or by performing different kinds of exercises. Then I would see additional weight loss or a decreased waistline.

Other measures of success can be how you feel—things that are harder to quantify, but equally important. For example, your energy level, your pain, your mood, your sleep patterns—these are more subjective but important nonetheless.

After a few months of improved eating habits, I had my annual physical. My cholesterol ratio improved. My LDL (bad) cholesterol decreased because I wasn't eating as much junk, and my HDL (good) cholesterol increased due to exercising. These results were very motivating. For years, I attributed my borderline cholesterol problem (slightly high bad cholesterol, too low good cholesterol) to genetics. It's true that genetic predisposition plays a role, but much of the problem was due to my own behaviors.

A whole new world opened up to me when I began to realize that lifestyle changes could have a positive impact on my health.

You might find that your blood pressure improves as you work on your exercise and eating goals. There are numerous health benefits associated with a normal-range Body Mass Index (BMI) and Waist-to-Hip Ratio (WHR), including decreased risk of diabetes and heart attacks, and certain cancers. Not only can your new, healthy lifestyle add real years to your life, but it can contribute towards a better quality of life.

I discovered that I had more stamina and didn't get out of breath as quickly when I exercised. I had more overall energy. I didn't feel as stressed. I wanted to do more, not less. I spent less time on the couch watching TV, and more time doing more purposeful activities that were good for my body and mind.

After a few months of slowly increasing the weights I was exercising with, I realized that I was stronger than when I first started. I asked Allan what he thought of those hard, unfamiliar areas that I began to notice on my arms and thighs. I thought it was a sign of some dreadful disease. He pointed out that those hard areas were muscles. Muscles? I have muscles?! Well, I guess they were always there, waiting to blossom and emerge in all their glory from beneath the layers of fat. That reminded me of a beautiful image from the poem *Ode to the West Wind* by Percy Bysshe Shelley (1819), "The winged seeds, where they lie cold and low/Each like a corpse within its grave, until/ Thine azure sister of the Spring shall blow" (7-9).

Yes, after a long winter of over 40 years, my muscles were emerging. My arms started to look strong and shapely as my excess fat began to disappear. My spare tire was becoming deflated and I could easily zip up my pants. Many of my clothes were literally falling off of me. A bathing suit I'd purchased six months prior was too loose. I had not worn a bikini in years, but I decided to go for it.

Sure, I wasn't perfect. I wasn't going to be recruited for a sports magazine's swimsuit model edition, but I felt great.

Of course, leave it to children to keep your ego in check. One day my eight-year-old son Joshua said, "Mummy, you look good. Your stomach is only half as fat as it used to be." Out of the mouths of babes.

It was now the end of June. I went to a swimwear shop to buy a bikini. I hadn't worn one in a decade, since before having children. In the past decade, I'd worn either a one-piece bathing suit, or a tankini which covered most of my abdomen.

I was delighted as I tried on several bikinis and they actually fit me in a size small for the bottom and medium for the top. The teenage salesgirls were not only encouraging and supportive, but they tried to convince me to try on the skimpiest of bikinis. Well, I know my limits. After all, a 44-year-old should not wear a bikini bottom so small that "Made in China" takes up half of the fabric. I went for a couple of sexy bikinis that provided tasteful coverage. This was the first time in memory that I had a positive experience buying swimsuits.

What should you do if you find that there are obstacles that are preventing you from accomplishing your goals? The two most common obstacles are lack of time and lack of motivation. There's also lack of money, for example, lack of money to buy healthier food or to purchase gear or to pay for a gym membership or a trainer. There's lack of encouragement and support from your spouse, partner, or other close family members and friends. There's lack of confidence. Inhibitions. Too busy. Too tired. Too lazy. There's fear of failure, fear of the unknown, and even fear of success. The list is endless. Everyone can find one or more reasons why they can't prepare healthy meals or do some exercise.

Another secret of success is to seek solutions! In the business world, when a problem arises on a project, an effective project manager finds workarounds and has contingency plans. You're the manager of your project to get fit and to improve your health. There are no excuses. Whether your obstacles are real or perceived, you must find ways to overcome them—even if it's inconvenient!

Some popular techniques used in sports psychology to deal with psychological hurdles include visualization and positive self-talk. Perhaps you're afraid to try something new because you're afraid you'll look foolish. You may be afraid to commit. Maybe you're anxious or you have low self-esteem.

Visualization involves imagining the desired outcome and picturing it in your mind. You can hone your creative skills by employing all of your imaginary senses. Imagine how you'll look and feel physically and mentally when you achieve your goal in a few months. Take, for example, my goal of running the tough hills from my cottage to the mailbox and back, a distance of about 8 kilometers. At first those hills seemed daunting and when I tried, it was really hard. Instead of giving up, I visualized how I'd feel when I completed that challenge. I never told myself, "*If* I complete it." I always said, "*When* I complete it." We have to cast doubts from our minds. This can be difficult especially if our new goals are in unfamiliar domains—ones we've never attempted before. That's where training our brains comes in. With lots of practice over an extended period of time, we can teach ourselves to overcome negative thoughts. Remember the little engine that could? He kept telling himself, "I think I can. I think I can." He didn't give up and eventually achieved his goal.

You can use positive self-talk, even a mantra, to change your inner dialogue. Your mantra can become your self-fulfilling prophecy. If you remind yourself in times of doubt, "I think I can," then you can.

What if your obstacles are real, not just a negative idea in your mind? For example, you don't think you have enough money to sign up for a fitness class or to purchase some personal training sessions. If you go through your budget and carefully analyze it, you may find you can cut back on some non-essentials.

You have to decide what your priorities and values are. If you're eating in restaurants, going to the movies, or your hobby is shopping, then you have to figure out what benefits you'll get from those activities compared with spending some of that money on your health. Look beyond the moment. What tangible benefits can you get from buying another pair of shoes, compared with spending that money on experts or gear that will help you get closer to your goals? Which choice will contribute to a better quality of life?

If you truly have financial hardships, look for activities that don't cost money. There are many fitness activities you can do for free or next to nothing. Look around and give it some thought. All the resources you need to succeed are out there waiting for you to embrace them. Don't be afraid to ask around. If you don't ask, you won't know. Walking, jogging, swimming in a public pool, or riding a bike are a few ideas. Some yoga studios periodically offer a free class to the public. Some public tennis courts are free of charge during off hours. Some non-profit organizations offer free fitness classes for people with low incomes or tight budgets. Seek and you shall find.

What if you don't have time? You have to schedule in your workouts and stick to those appointments, just as you would do for important business meetings or medical appointments.

If pain is your obstacle, avoiding exercise is not the answer. If you give up on exercise, you miss out on all the health benefits. Find out from your doctor or a fitness professional what exercise is suitable for your condition. Many chronic pain sufferers benefit from aquatic exercise classes because being up to your waist or shoulders in water reduces much of the load on your joints. A personal trainer can assess you and create an exercise program that is modified to address your physical issues.

Another common obstacle is the need for childcare. I see many parents out walking or jogging with their babies and toddlers in strollers, or cycling with their children in child seats. There are even fitness classes designed for new parents and their babies. Some training facilities offer childcare at a nominal cost. Find a friend and take turns babysitting for each other so you can get some exercise.

Cultural and religious barriers may be your obstacles. For example, your religious beliefs may not allow you to be seen by the opposite sex engaging in exercise or wearing clothing that doesn't meet your religious standards of modesty. That could mean you can't exercise in a gym or community center, you can't swim in a public pool, or you can't go jogging in a T-shirt and shorts. In such cases, solutions may include working out in a private studio with a personal trainer of the same gender, or exercising in the privacy of your home with a workout video.

If you stop telling yourself "I can't because…" and replace that with "I can because…," you'll come up with practical solutions to your problems. When I stopped focusing on obstacles and making excuses, when I learned to jump over hurdles rather than stop dead in my tracks in front of them, and when I made up my mind that I was going to achieve my goals no matter what, I figured out how. When I opened my mind to success, I was able to see solutions that were in front of me all along. When you're truly committed to achieving your goals, nothing will stop you.

Gloria Schwartz

Personal Best Exercises

o   List one or more short-term goals and the criteria you will use to measure and evaluate your success with each goal.

o   List one or more long-term goals and evaluation criteria.

o   List any obstacles that stand between you and your goals, and then write realistic strategies for overcoming these obstacles.

Did you know?

•   Short- and long-term goals should be difficult and challenging, but realistic. You should feel you can achieve them in a reasonable amount of time based on your current abilities.

•   Short-term goals can be stepping stones to long-term goals.

•   Limiting the number of goals you set and then prioritizing them helps you determine where to focus your efforts.

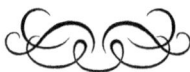

4 FOOD

I had to learn over time how to shift my thoughts and behaviors.

What do you really eat? Why are you overweight? It all boils down to input and output. To lose weight, you must create a caloric deficit. That means you must eat fewer calories than you use, so your body is getting some energy from its fat storage cells.

Almost everyone I know has been on a diet. Diets don't work. Diets are unrealistic. Diets are not satisfying. They leave you feeling hungry and irritable. You can't stay on a diet forever. Diet is a four-letter word. Don't be fooled by the exaggerated claims and celebrity endorsements that the multi-billion-dollar diet industry employs to drive sales. Forget about fad diets. Diets offer false hope based on faulty premises. The current diet trend, as evidenced by the plethora of best-selling diet books, is to vilify a single nutrient, particular foods, or an entire food group. For example, eliminating carbohydrates may promote initial weight loss; however, your body needs carbs. They provide you with a significant source of energy.

Diets have catchy names and are promoted as offering a "breakthrough," but they are really just different combinations of fat, protein, and carbohydrates. There are negligible differences between all of these diets. Most people initially lose weight and most of the lost weight is regained.

You need a healthy balance of macronutrients (carbohydrates, protein, and fats) for energy, and essential micronutrients (vitamins and minerals). Complex carbs, lean protein, and healthy fats are best.

You should eat a variety of healthy foods every day and eat an amount that's appropriate for your age, height, weight, gender, and activity level. If you eat too few calories, your body wants to hang on to the fat, not shed it, as it thinks there's a famine. Diets based on regimented eating plans or too few calories are not sustainable. Extreme caloric restriction can be damaging to your body.

Diet companies that sell prepackaged meals or meal-replacement shakes may convince you they're giving you a jumpstart, but they are actually profiting off of your dependency and fail to teach life skills necessary for long-term success. Those diets are selling a lifestyle of convenience, not a lifestyle of health. Many of the ready-made meals and snacks promoted on diet infomercials and commercials are appealing treats like cake and burgers. You're wowed with incredible before-and-after photos and assured that you can "eat all that *and* lose weight!" Yes, you *can* lose weight with those calorically-reduced diet programs, but they typically fail to provide the right nourishment for your bodies and, like most diets, they're difficult to adhere to. Most of these shakes, bars, and other so-called weight-loss food products contain unhealthy ingredients such as fructose and palm oil, or other lesser-known man-made ingredients that are difficult to pronounce and not found in nature. That's not a healthy way to eat.

Some companies that sell shakes claim on their websites that they offer health and wealth. They basically want you to become an associate and sell their products, which is how they get rich. This cash-cow philosophy would definitely get me exercising—I'd run as fast as possible in the opposite direction!

You should also be skeptical of cleanses, herbal diets, supplements, or other products and alternative therapies claiming to detoxify your body. Just because your favorite actor is doing it, that doesn't mean it works. Your body is designed to naturally and efficiently remove what it doesn't need through your liver, kidneys, and colon. Be wary of the communal reinforcement phenomenon— that's the process by which a claim becomes widely believed through repetition even if it has not been properly researched and has no empirical data to support it. Don't be fooled by pseudo-science, fear-mongering, artificial creation of a need when the need doesn't exist, or anecdotal information such as customer success stories. There's a reason why these products have no legitimate science to back up their claims. At best, a detox is a symbolic, but unnecessary, act that may represent a new start. Without significant lifestyle changes, it's pointless.

Fads such as gluten-free diets are not only unnecessary (unless you've been medically diagnosed with Celiac disease), but they are misleading on several levels. Cutting out grains containing gluten can lead to a nutritional deficiency. Why risk that if it's not medically necessary? Look at all the gluten-free processed foods that have flooded the market. And they're expensive. So many people suddenly believe they're sensitive to gluten and are jumping on the bandwagon. The medical profession has come up with a name that refers to the phenomenon when sufferers of Irritable Bowel Syndrome or other digestive issues feel better on a gluten-free diet: Non-Celiac Gluten Sensitivity. But these sufferers may feel the same improvements or better on a low FODMAP[1] diet, which suggests it's actually some types of carbohydrates and not the protein gluten, that they have difficulty digesting.

If going gluten-free reduces your cramps, bloating, burping, diarrhea, or constipation, that's great. Feeling more energetic or happier may be due to the placebo effect or to weight loss that results from eliminating processed foods containing gluten or cutting back on overall calories. Caveat emptor! Gluten-free cake mixes, cookies, and sugary breakfast cereals are not healthy even though they're sold at health food stores. These products are targeted not just at sufferers of Celiac disease, but to everyone, which is why they're also sold at mainstream grocery stores. The manufacturers are looking at their bottom line and have managed to convince consumers that a gluten-free diet is the panacea for a wide range of problems. In fact, health issues are often multifactorial. Some people who go on a gluten-free diet simply to lose weight actually gain weight because many gluten-free processed foods are high in calories. If you do not have Celiac disease and you want to lose weight and get healthier, instead of going gluten-free, go glutton-free!

With any type of diet, the vast majority of dieters who lose weight gain it back—plus extra weight—as soon as they stop dieting

---

[1]FODMAP stands for Fermentable Oligo-Di-Mono-saccharides And Polyols. A low FODMAP diet limits consumption of these nutrients which occur naturally in some whole foods. FODMAP foods include those containing fructose (fruit, honey, corn syrup), lactose (dairy), fructans/inulin (e.g., wheat, onion, garlic), galactans (e.g., beans, lentils, legumes), and polyols (artificial sweeteners and fruits containing pits).

and return to their normal eating habits. While you're likely to lose weight on a strict diet protocol, it's nearly impossible to maintain that lifestyle long-term without compromising your health. The diet industry is designed to set you up for short-term success and long-term failure—it makes billions of dollars on return customers seeking the latest diet.

You'll get better results with your weight and health if you learn how to eat sensibly—and stick with it! Sustainable lifestyle choices offer a better chance of long-term weight management.

You'll have more long-term success if you adopt some or all of the following lifestyle strategies, which you can phase in over time:

- Increase your consumption of fruits and vegetables, and the frequency, intensity, and duration of physical activity

- Decrease the overall calories, unhealthy fats, sweets and junk food you consume, and decrease your portion sizes

⚭

Many of us consume far too much added sugar. The American Heart Association recommends no more than nine teaspoons per day for men and six for women. Most processed foods contain added sugar, even those which we wouldn't expect, such as yogurt, pasta sauce, bread, and peanut butter. Sugar can be addictive. It triggers the release of dopamine and gives us a euphoric feeling. Some research suggests sugar is as addictive as cocaine.

Eating fruit and other whole foods that naturally contain sugar is different than eating added sugar because the former provide micronutrients and fiber. Added sugar has no nutritional benefits. It's better to eat a piece of fruit than a glass of juice because you'll feel satiated more easily. The juicing trend, especially when juicing fruits, is not the best approach. It's so easy to drink too many calories and lots of sugar. Tooth decay is associated with overconsumption of both added and natural sugars. Excess sugar consumption is also associated with weight gain, type 2 diabetes, cardiovascular disease, certain cancers, and non-alcoholic fatty liver disease.

You have to be a detective to figure out when sugar is added. It may be listed as fructose, glucose, sucrose, maltose, dextrose, lactose, high fructose corn syrup, cane juice, agave, or other names.

My plan is not about perfection. It's about improvement. It's not rocket science. You get fat by eating too much food that you're not burning off. The excess energy gets stored in your body as fat. Your body cannot enjoy optimum health and vigor unless you nourish it with high-quality food in appropriate amounts on a regular basis. We only get one body, yet so many of us neglect it. It's never too late to change. You can right-size your body and improve your health at any age and at any stage of life.

Nutrition labels, food advertisements, and commercials can be misleading, even downright deceptive. When a food product is labelled as "reduced fat" or "low sodium," it is often a marketing gimmick. What is deemed "low sodium" may seem low if you think eating a truckload of salt per day is normal. What is sold as "reduced fat" may be reduced compared to a former version of the product, but it may still be high in fat. "Low fat" is a sneaky marketing term. These products often have extra sugar to make them palatable. Since the market was inundated with low-fat products a few decades ago, more people have become overweight and obese.

In Canada, food manufacturers can pay for the right to print a national health foundation's logo on their products. Talk about conflict of interest! Different versions of the same product, one with no added sodium, the other containing a significant amount of sodium per serving, can both have the logo. Some sugar-laden foods have received this logo as well, implying that such products are good for you. Put on your consumer's flak jacket. The supermarket is a minefield! How's the average person supposed to decipher labels with all this confusing and misleading information?

Let's examine a granola bar to see if it's low fat. People think granola bars are healthy. Most granola bars actually have a caloric content and nutritional value similar to a chocolate bar. Suppose a granola bar has 140 calories and 5 grams of fat. That doesn't sound bad. Now, let's dig a bit deeper. Fat is very dense in calories. Each gram of fat contains nine calories (compared to just 4 calories in a gram of protein and 4 calories in a gram of carbohydrates). To calculate the percentage of fat, multiply the grams of fat in the serving size by 9. Divide the number by the total calories per serving. In the granola bar example, 5 grams of fat times 9 equals 45. Forty-five divided by 140 calories is .32. That means 32 percent of the calories you're eating in that granola bar comes from fat. Is that item low fat? Absolutely not! In general, we should be getting between 20 and 30 percent of our calories from fat, and not just any kind of fat, but healthy fats from oily fish, nuts, seeds, and some oils. If you read the nutritional information on a granola bar package, you'll see that some of the fat is saturated. That's the unhealthy kind of fat that contributes to weight gain and heart disease. If you consume high amounts of unhealthy fats on a regular basis, then you're potentially causing damage to your body. You want healthy food—including healthy types of fat in suitable quantities—to fuel your body.

A basic knowledge of how to read food labels will help you make better choices. Just because a product is marketed as a healthy choice, that does not make it so.

⤲⟐⤳

As part of the blueprint, I recommend that you start keeping a detailed food journal for up to seven days. Be honest and record everything—and I mean *everything*—that you eat and drink. It's easy to fool yourself and mask your real eating habits with improved eating if you only keep a journal for a day or two.

Many studies have shown that a food journal is an effective tool for weight loss because it increases your awareness. Some of my clients discount the idea of keeping a food journal. They already know what they eat, or so they claim as soon as I suggest the journal-keeping exercise; but when I query them about what they ate the previous day or even the same morning, they can't remember. When you record everything you consume, you become aware and accountable. The act of self-monitoring forces you to consider what you're putting in your mouth. Keeping a journal long-term will help more. Don't use the excuse that you don't have time to keep a food journal. It takes a few minutes per day. If something is important to you, you'll make time. If you're tech savvy, use an app to save time.

We tend to underestimate the amount of food that we eat. When you examine your food journal, you'll see the truth and you'll likely uncover patterns. If you're lost, show it to a personal trainer or a dietician. They can help you identify areas for improvement.

Here's a sample of a basic food journal with some fictitious entries. You can include more details if you like, for example, calories consumed, and your emotions and activities while eating (e.g., bored, stressed, watching TV, driving, dining with friends).

Day/ Date	Time	Meal/ Snack	Details
Mon. May 1	7 a.m.	breakfast	2 eggs, 1 bagel with jam and butter, coffee with cream and sugar
	10 a.m.	snack	coffee with cream and sugar, 1 blueberry muffin
	12 p.m.	lunch	1 slice pizza, 1 can diet cola, 1 apple
	2 p.m.	snack	1 chocolate bar, water
	6:15 p.m.	dinner	6 ounces grilled chicken, 1 slice bread and butter, green salad, apple pie, tea
	8:30 p.m.	snack	1 banana, 1 cup homogenized milk
	10 p.m.	Snack	1 can diet soda, half of a family-size bag of chips

Some of the poor habits that jump out of this sample food journal are the over-consumption of simple carbohydrates and high-fat dairy products. Soda and coffee are the beverages of choice rather than water. There's an insufficient consumption of fresh produce. There's late-night snacking on empty calories.

Once you've identified your own dietary weak spots, list some unhealthy foods you commonly eat that you're willing to eliminate or at least reduce. In addition, list a few healthy foods that you don't normally eat and that you're willing to introduce. You need to learn how to eat intelligently. You must actively consider the consequences of each decision. Will that slice of pizza help you achieve your goals?

If you're overweight, then you're probably an overeater. That means you consume more calories than you burn. It's important to understand *why* you overeat and *why* you make unhealthy choices. Are you unhappy, anxious, depressed, bored, or lonely? When you figure out the underlying reasons for your poor eating habits, you can work at finding solutions. If you're trying to fill a void by comforting yourself with food, find a more productive way to fill it. If you can't figure out the *why* behind your eating issues, seek professional help.

❧❧❧

I used to hang around with a friend who happened to be very slim. We once went to see a movie together. I ordered popcorn and a soda. She had nothing during the movie. I felt like a pig as I munched my popcorn that was swimming in buttery topping and I slurped my soda, while she happily enjoyed the movie without a snack. I never went to the movies with her again. I felt like she put a damper on my fun even though she didn't comment on what I was eating or drinking. I felt guilty. It was only years later that I realized she was wise. Why did I need junk food to enjoy the movie? I wasn't really hungry at the time; it was just a learned habit, something I always did when I went to the movies. Not that I go to the movies that often, so why worry? Well, I watch TV every day and that same habit applied to my TV viewing. I never sat down with a bowl of spinach to watch a show. It was a bag of chips or a bowl of popcorn or a handful or cookies or all of those things.

Bad habits—you've got to break them. You've got to get it into your mind that when you go to a movie or anywhere else, you don't have to have junk food to enjoy the experience. Yes, you can have it, but it's not necessary. Now when I go to a movie, I buy (or more typically, smuggle in my purse) a bottle of water to drink during the show. I either bring a healthy snack, buy a small bag of plain popcorn as a treat, or eat nothing at all. Boo for me, right? What a pathetic person you think I am right now! That's because you're not living a healthy lifestyle. You've got to learn to think like a champion!

I used to be a glutton. I didn't eat huge meals, but I ate tons of junk. I ate with little regard for my health. My body responded accordingly by slowly gaining weight—that was the visible damage. The more disconcerting damage was on the inside.

Make no mistake about it: If you're overweight, it's probably because you eat too much of the wrong things and you don't move enough.

I can't stand it when heavy people tell me that they hardly eat. Let's get real. We don't get overweight by breathing too much fresh air. When I was overweight, it was because of my lifestyle choices.

Overweight people may lie about what they eat, or they are in denial. Many are unaware of the excessive quantity and the poor quality of the foods they eat. What may seem like an appropriate meal to one person may actually be an abnormally large portion with an excessive caloric content for their body size and activity level. Many people simply don't know what moderation looks like.

Please don't use the genetics card with me. You can fool yourself into blaming genetics. Lots of people say, "My mom was fat. My dad was fat. I'm fat. So it's genetic." Did you ever consider that your parents may have been fat because of their lifestyle, that they taught you poor eating habits, and were poor role models? There are very few people who are actually fat because of genetics, perhaps five percent. Currently, more than two-thirds of North American adults are overweight or obese. Pre-diabetes and type 2 diabetes are rampant. Obesity now poses a greater global health threat than malnutrition! In most parts of the world, more young adults are dying from non-communicable diseases, such as heart disease and cancer, than from starvation or communicable diseases. The culprit is the Western lifestyle that the majority of countries have adopted. Essentially, we are eating ourselves to death. Clearly, genetics doesn't play much of a role, if any, in the vast majority of cases. Even if you are genetically predisposed to gain weight or hang on to it, much of that can be overcome with a healthier lifestyle. You have the power to break the cycle of obesity.

You can't always judge a book by its cover. It's not just overweight or obese people who have health problems or risks. One in four thin adults has high blood pressure, high blood glucose (sugar), and abnormal levels of cholesterol. "Normal-weight obesity" or "skinny-fat" are terms used to describe people who are of normal weight or have a Body Mass Index of under 25 and who don't have a lot of adipose tissue—the kind of fat you can see and pinch—but have a high amount of visceral or internal body fat. Visceral fat is dangerous because it's deep inside the abdomen and surrounds the organs. Like their obese counterparts, skinny-fat people are at an increased risk for disease.

Some overweight people attribute their weight issues to hypothyroidism (low thyroid hormone production). I've heard many people claim that they must have a thyroid problem or a slow metabolism because they seem to gain weight easily or have difficulty losing weight. A small percentage of people have hypothyroidism. It's more common in women than men, and its incidence increases with age. A diagnosis and prescription can resolve this medical condition and help with weight-related symptoms; however, if you continue over-eating and don't burn off excess calories with physical activity, a pill that fixes hypothyroidism won't completely fix your weight problem. The obesity epidemic cannot be explained by hypothyroidism, which, like genetics, is an excuse some individuals use rather than examining their lifestyle.

The scientific theories about the cause of obesity are, at present, inconclusive. Obesity may be caused by excessive overeating that some people require to satisfy the brain's pleasure center to the same degree that lean people experience from less food. Some modern foods that are dense in fat and sugar and look appetizing can affect the brain's reward system and override the appetite-suppressing hormones such that it's difficult to control consumption.

∽৩৩৵

I'm not here to tell you exactly what to eat. I'm not promoting a diet. I've intentionally never even been on a diet. I want you to think *lifestyle*. Lifestyle is something you can change slowly over time, not overnight. Incremental changes to what and how you eat, how you think about food, when you eat, how often you eat, where you eat, why you eat, the quality of the food that you eat—these are things you can realistically and successfully accomplish and maintain, regardless of your weight, age, or gender.

Food is necessary for life. Food is supposed to be your friend. It is your fuel. If you abuse food, it becomes your foe. Eating when you're not hungry, binge eating, regularly putting calorie-dense, nutritionally-depleted junk into your body, developing food addictions or disordered eating, and consuming more calories than you burn are just some of the symptoms of a toxic relationship with food. Food addictions can manifest in different ways, to different degrees. In order to overcome an addiction, you have to admit to it.

Unlike an alcoholic who can potentially learn to stop drinking alcohol, human beings can't stop eating. We need to eat to live. That's why we need to learn to eat right.

Food contributes towards as much as 80% of your body weight.

Physical activity contributes 10 to 15%. Depending on the source, you may find slightly different figures, but it's generally agreed that food is a major player and genetic factors contribute only about 5% towards weight. You can blame genes on some of your problems, but you have the power to control up to 95% of contributing factors through your choices and actions.

The gene pool remains fairly stable for generations. Therefore, it's not our change in genes, as a population, that's caused an obesity epidemic in the last few decades. It's the change in our environment that has greatly influenced our behavior—how we eat and the amount of physical activity we get. Even if you are in the small minority of people with a genetic predisposition to obesity, you can counteract gene-related risks with a healthy lifestyle. Our genes are not our destiny. Most people who have the "obesity genes" do not become overweight or obese.

It takes 3500 excess calories to gain a pound of fat. If you consistently consume 500 more calories per day than you burn—which is not that difficult to do—you'll gain a pound per week. You can do the math and figure out how many pounds you'd gain in a year. In case you're not good at math, here's the answer: 52 pounds! That extra chocolate bar, a few crackers with peanut butter, those chips, the sodas, the larger portions—they all add up over time.

In addition to the quantity of food and calories, there are different qualities of input for you to take into consideration. Your body needs high-quality, nutrient-dense calories. You can eat generous quantities of food without getting fat if you make healthy choices. Oftentimes, people think what they are eating is healthy when it's not. If a processed food has numerous ingredients and many of them are hard to pronounce, then it's likely that it's bad for you, or at least not an optimal choice. Whole natural foods such as a fruit, a vegetable, a lean piece of grilled or steamed protein like turkey, fish or chicken—these are examples of good choices. Fruit-flavored snacks, fries, and fried chicken fingers—poor choices. And just because a diet soda has zero calories, that doesn't make it a healthy choice. Water is the ultimate beverage. Our bodies need it.

⋘⋙

At my peak weight of 157, I admitted to myself that food had become a struggle. At 5 feet 5 inches tall, I was overweight. More important than the numbers, my body consisted of a high proportion of fat and a low proportion of muscle, and I was unfit. I was on a self-destructive path that would undoubtedly lead to a heavier body and more health problems if I didn't change my ways.

I loved junk and I loved convenience. Period. I'd been that way all my adult life. I was never into drugs or booze. But I couldn't eat just one cookie. I couldn't have just a couple of chips. If I brought junk food into my house, it had to get out of my house, via my colon. I'd buy a bag of cookies for my children, and when they went to sleep, I'd eat not one or two, but easily five or more. Okay, full disclosure—10 or more! It was as if the cookies had voices. I'd be watching TV, when all of a sudden I swear I could hear Chocolate Chip calling my name from the kitchen cupboard, "Gloria, I'm waiting for you." How enticing. I could never resist. I'd tell myself that I'd have just one more cookie, but I was fooling myself. Several trips to the kitchen later, the bag was empty. I thought I had a sweet tooth. In retrospect, I was a binge eater, not in the clinical sense where people can binge on 5000 or more calories in one sitting, but in the sense that I had episodes where I couldn't resist over-indulging on sweet or salty snacks even when I wasn't hungry.

"Mummy, where are all the cookies?" my son Jesse would ask the next day as he shook the empty bag upside down.

Addictions can be a lifelong struggle. As I improved my eating habits, I still allowed myself to indulge in treats to satisfy my cravings. However, I realized that the less often and the smaller amounts of treats I had, the less I craved them. Willpower came into play. I had to actively force myself to say "No!" to the temptations that surrounded me: the drive-thru that's on nearly every corner; the chocolate bars next to every store's checkout; and the TV commercials that tried to seduce me into ordering pizza or buying sugary, salty, and fatty snacks.

Addiction and willpower. The devil and the angel. Don't we all experience competing thoughts at times? We feel like we're being pushed and pulled in different directions from within. Do we give in to impulses that give us instant gratification, or do we choose healthier actions that provide delayed gratification?

I had to learn how to consciously shift and shape my thoughts and behaviors—essentially, retrain my brain. I'll be honest with you. I continue to this day to have treats, perhaps a few too many. I never set the expectation that I or anyone should eat "perfectly." That would be unrealistic and anxiety-provoking for most people, including myself. I feel I have significantly improved. For me, that's good enough. Let me clarify what I mean by good enough. Good enough means I'm proud of how far I've come. Good enough is a moving target. I continue to work at making good enough better.

⁂

Did you ever eat a banana or an apple that had to be fortified with vitamins? No. They're perfectly healthy in their natural state. That's how we should eat. Pizza, for example, contains over-processed white flour crust and loads of high-fat and high-sodium cheese. A single slice of pizza from popular restaurant chains contains between 200 and 900 milligrams of sodium. Let's be honest. Few of us stop at one slice. If you have a few slices, you may have consumed more sodium in one sitting than your recommended daily allowance. That's not heart-healthy. Not to mention the artery-clogging fat in the cheese and greasy meat toppings. Like most dishes, pizza can be a decent meal if you prepare it yourself with better ingredients.

I had lots of bad habits that were difficult to overcome. I loved convenience foods, I loved snacking, and I loved eating out. I'd eat out several times per week! It was a way to socialize and more importantly, it was easy. Allan and I would have a date night once a week, which typically involved going out for dinner. On the weekends, we'd take the kids out for a fast-food lunch. We could easily keep our children placated with plastic toys and fries while we scoffed down burgers, fries, and diet soft drinks. The calorie-free diet drinks seemed to justify everything. An ice cream sundae would often round out the meal. Then Allan and I would sit like snakes with full bellies while our sons ran around in the indoor play area. Even though we ate lunch out, we'd often take the kids out again for dinner. Because the boys were young, we chose family-style restaurants—where quantity and affordability take precedence over quality.

All of this eating out seemed normal to us. Many of our friends ate out frequently. Birds of a feather flock together. We were

45

entrenched in a culture of convenience. We'd been sucked into the vortex of complacency and brainwashed by advertising into thinking that there was no harm in eating this way.

During those years when I was eating like that, I rarely inquired about nutritional information. I never thought about the bad habits I was teaching my children, and I was oblivious to the long-term health implications for myself and my family. I had no interest in knowing. In hindsight, I was in the Pre-contemplation stage of readiness for change. I was not at all ready! I can tell you now, based on the current information on the website for that regularly-frequented fast-food chain, that I was consuming 1230 calories, 1684 milligrams of sodium, 60 grams of fat (21 saturated), and 14 teaspoons of sugar—all in a single meal! Those figures are extremely high.

Work meant junk food as well. Co-workers often brought donuts or muffins to the office. Departmental work lunches were catered. We were served deli sandwiches or pizza with sodas and chips. Overall, it was a culture of bad eating. I rarely resisted the temptations. I admit that I was often the ringleader who'd round up my work friends for a lunch outing. We typically went for fast food since we had to be back at the office in under an hour. These outings happened a few times per week for years. Again, I would convince myself that I wasn't eating badly if I had a diet drink or if I skipped the fries. It was years later that I became aware of all the salt, calories, and fat hidden in even the most innocuous looking burger. Even though a diet soda isn't fattening, it's garbage that I was intentionally putting into my body. Definitely not good for my kidneys. The sugary taste of the artificial sweeteners in the diet sodas had me hooked like a crack addict. The more soda I drank, the more I craved. I typically drank leading brand colas, often a couple of cans per day—maybe more. It's now been five years since I gave up drinking soda. Based on my conservative estimate of two cans per day, if I hadn't quit that habit, I would have drunk at least 3,650 cans of soda in the past five years. That's over 5 bathtubs full!

When I wasn't eating out, supper at home often meant throwing a frozen, store-bought lasagne or some other convenience food into the oven after a long day at work. It was definitely easy. Allan and I were often too tired or too lazy to cook a proper meal or to prepare something the night before. Our kids liked these kinds of fiber-free, easy-to-swallow foods, which meant less coaxing, begging, cajoling, screaming, crying, and fighting at the dinner table. Of course, we all know what happens when you live on a low fiber diet—constipation. Once I changed my lifestyle, that problem resolved itself.

One day I saw an episode of the Canadian TV show *Marketplace* that exposed the nutritional information for many menu items at several popular family-style restaurants. The amount of salt, fat, and calories was incredible. I hadn't realized, since such information is not readily available at most restaurants, just how bad nearly every menu item is. Even items promoted as "healthy choices" were often over-sized portions with high fat content, tons of sodium, and many more calories than I would consume if I made a similar meal at home from scratch. It was at that moment that a light bulb went off in my head!

When the episode ended, I excitedly emailed several friends and shared what I had learned. It was then, too, that I made a decision to significantly reduce the number of meals I would eat out. I also vowed to be more selective with the types of restaurants I visited, and to cook more meals rather than serve convenience foods.

Fast forward to 2013. I was featured in a viewer feedback segment on that same TV show *Marketplace*. I described how that episode, years earlier, had impacted my life and how I'd transformed my mind and body. The show was seen by viewers across Canada and was replayed numerous times during the year. It was an unexpected opportunity for me to share my important message. I was living proof that small changes yield big results.

That one decision—to improve my eating habits—not only impacted me, it impacted my family. Initially, Allan and our sons were upset with me when I told them I didn't want to eat out anymore, or at least not more than once every week or two. Allan would suggest going out for lunch or dinner on the weekend, and when I'd say no, he would complain and try to dissuade me. That only aggravated me.

"You're trying to sabotage me," I'd bark accusingly.

"Oh Mummy," whined Jesse and Joshua, rolling their eyes. I'd tell the three of them to go out without me. I'd eat at home. At first they went without me, but after a few times, they didn't want to do that.

I did most of the grocery shopping so I typically controlled what came into the house. After a few weeks of complaining and whining, we settled into a pattern of eating at home rather than running to restaurants. If we were out shopping, I'd plan to go home for lunch rather than grab a quick bite at the mall; or, I'd ensure we ate at home first. Bringing a few snacks, like some fruit and bottled water, was always a good plan. That helped us all resist temptations and stave off hunger pangs. For the times that we did eat out, I tried really hard to select the best of the worst; that is, foods that were not fried, had no sauces, and had lots of veggies, and I'd request that no salt be added. Of course, many restaurants pre-season their food with salt since it's a cheaper alternative to using better cuts of meat or seasoning with fresh herbs; at least I was trying to make informed choices. I'd go as far as to check the restaurant's website for nutritional information. If it was available, I'd make my menu selection in advance.

Jesse and Joshua began to adopt some of my new habits. It seemed most challenging for Allan. I'd question his choices to get him to think twice, which more often than not resulted in him making a healthier choice. After a couple of months, he told me his pants were feeling loose around the waist.

"And why do you think that is?" I asked smugly. "It's because I haven't been buying junk food for the house and we hardly eat out anymore," I blurted out before he had a chance to respond. He had to admit that I was right.

Imagine how much more we could improve ourselves inside and out if we made a few additional changes here and there to our lifestyles, I thought to myself. And so, the loose pants that hung from our waists motivated me to seek out more ways to improve.

One step I decided to take was to keep a food journal for self-assessment purposes. I scrutinized my entries and became increasingly aware of my patterns. This helped me decide what types of foods to add to my diet and what to remove or decrease. I also got a better understanding of when and why I was eating.

I became acutely aware that I needed something in my system every day before leaving the house, even if it was just a small meal. For much of my adult life, breakfast had consisted of a donut or a salt-laden egg-and-cheese on an English muffin that I picked up at the drive-thru on my way to the office. Now I was learning to sit down at the kitchen table and have something to last me for the first part of the morning. I had always ensured my children ate breakfast before they went to school. Now I was practicing what I preached. I also wanted to be a better role model.

I noticed through my journal entries that I wasn't eating often enough. What I needed to do was have a healthy snack mid-morning and mid-afternoon and even a little something in the evening, something nutritious to fill me up and help me resist impulse eating and poor choices. I learned that if you eat five to six smaller meals per day—rather than three square meals—you feel more satiated and you can better control blood glucose and hence, cravings.

I increasingly worked at cutting back on processed food. I was making more informed decisions. I had read a very eye-opening book entitled *Twinkie Deconstructed* (2008) that described in graphic detail the origin and manipulation of many common ingredients in processed food. For example, I learned that "natural colors" and "natural flavors" are actually created in a lab, often contain chemicals, and do not resemble anything found in nature. Now I was looking beyond trans fats, sodium, and calories per serving. I was also avoiding products that contained anything with the word "modified" in them. Thus, the processed foods that I now deemed acceptable were very few and far between.

I haven't yet leaped into the world of organic food, simply because my local grocery stores carry a very limited and over-priced range of such items. Perhaps organic food will become more widely available and affordable in the coming years. Even though organic food does not have significant nutritional advantages over conventionally-produced food, all those pesticides, growth hormones, and antibiotics in non-organic food can't be good for us.

By taking an honest look at what I was consuming and under what circumstances, I was able to revise the way I dealt with food. Once I weaned myself off of junk food, the cravings subsided, and I eventually felt physically better with improved eating habits. Gluttony is no longer a problem—at least not for the most part. But I never claimed that I am perfect. Perfection is highly over-rated. If I were perfect, I'd have nothing left to strive for!

Gloria Schwartz

Personal Best Exercises

o   Commit to keeping a food journal for one week.

o   Identify one unhealthy eating habit that you can eliminate completely or modify, beginning immediately. Identify one healthier eating habit that you can introduce immediately.

o   Put more thought and effort into meal planning and preparation rather than grabbing on the go. Educate yourself on portion control, how to choose more nutritious foods, and how to cook food in healthier ways. Spend time in the gym *and* the kitchen.

Did you know?

•   *When* we eat, not just *what* we eat, plays a role in weight loss. Our metabolism is influenced by our circadian rhythm—a 24-hour biological process. Disrupting your circadian rhythm, such as by working night shifts, can lead to weight gain.

•   People who have their biggest meal at breakfast eat less at dinner, and eat fewer evening snacks. They have more success with weight loss, as well as lower levels of insulin, glucose, and triglycerides throughout the day.

•   Vitamin and mineral supplements are useful when medically necessary. A blood test can determine if you have a deficiency. Taking supplements without your doctor's approval, such as herbal supplements or any supplements in high doses, can interfere with some medications or cause adverse side effects.

•   Not all calories are created equal. Our bodies use different amounts of energy to digest and process macronutrients. This is the Thermic Effect of Food (TEF). About 20 to 35% of calories consumed from protein get used processing it. The TEF for fats and carbs is 5 to 15%. Therefore, it's easier to gain weight eating candy than turkey, even if the calories are the same.

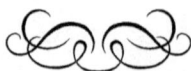

5 EXERCISE

I knew I had arrived at a new turning point in my transformation when I was upset that the gym would be closed on certain days.

Now we come to the exercise component of the blueprint. Exercise is essential. If you aren't in a physically demanding job, you need to add physical activities to your daily routine. Sitting is the new smoking. It's terrible for your health. Our bodies were designed to move. Technology has significantly reduced the amount of time we spend standing and doing natural movements like walking, lifting, pulling, and pushing.

The majority of people who exercise just want to lose weight and look good. The reality is that exercise plays a modest role in weight loss and weight management. So why should we exercise?

Exercise helps us get and stay fit. What is fitness? Fitness is not about a sexy-looking body, although that's what the diet and fitness industries tend to promote. Fitness is a physical and mental state that enhances your health. It's not just about *looking* healthy. You can remove fat from your thighs or abdomen with liposuction, but your new shape won't necessarily equate to improved internal health.

Exercise provides tremendous benefits for your physical and mental health. Exercise has been proven to reduce the risk of a wide variety of health issues including coronary heart disease, stroke, hypertension, breast cancer, colon cancer, osteoporosis, and type 2 diabetes. Exercise can also slow the progression of some diseases.

Just a few decades ago, people with cardiovascular disease or other ailments were discouraged by their doctors from exerting themselves; today, people in good health, as well as those with health issues, are encouraged to move and exercise.

Cardiorespiratory exercise, also known as cardio or aerobic exercise, develops your cardiorespiratory fitness, including strengthening your heart and increasing your lung capacity. Your heart is a muscle and needs to be exercised to remain healthy. Examples of cardio exercise are walking and stair climbing, which you can incorporate into your day-to-day life, and sports, such as running, cycling, and swimming. You can also get a cardio workout using a treadmill, an elliptical machine, or a stationary bike, or by taking different types of aerobics classes.

Heart disease is a leading cause of premature death in North American adults. You can reduce your risk of heart disease by engaging in cardio exercise. Cardio reduces hypertension, resting heart rate, and LDL (bad) cholesterol, and increases HDL (good) cholesterol.

Cardio is also beneficial because it burns fat, resulting in a leaner body which, in turn, reduces the risk of developing type 2 diabetes. Cardio increases energy and endurance, making sports as well as everyday activities less fatiguing. Cardio can also reduce the risk of certain cancers such as breast and colon cancer. It can lessen the symptoms of some chronic diseases such as arthritis. Some studies suggest that cardio may even prevent or delay the onset of Alzheimer's disease and dementia, and slow the progression of Parkinson's disease.

Cardio also benefits mental health by increasing levels of mood-enhancing brain chemicals. Going for a brisk walk or jog may lift your mood and alleviate anxiety, stress, and mild depression.

Resistance training, also known as strength training, develops your muscles and increases your strength. Examples of resistance training exercises are push-ups, pull-ups, and sit-ups. You can do resistance training using a variety of equipment such as dumbbells or machines, or using your own body weight.

Benefits of resistance training include an increase in lean muscle mass and an improved metabolism. Your body will become more efficient at burning fat and you'll even burn a few more calories while at rest. Another benefit is improved bone density, which lowers your risk for osteoporosis. Stronger muscles also improve your balance, posture, and coordination, thereby reducing your chance of falling and injuring yourself. Stronger muscles make everyday activities, such as lifting and carrying items, easier. Strength training is suitable for all ages. It should be done with moderate intensity for beginners. Once you have the right form (so you can prevent injuries), you can perform strength-training exercise with a higher intensity that is challenging, yet still takes into account any specific health issues and physical limitations. Performing a high number of repetitions with cute little dumbbells is a waste of time. You should put lots of effort into your workouts, exert yourself, and break a sweat.

Flexibility training, also called stretching, is often neglected. Stretching is important for several reasons. It can increase flexibility and help with mobility. It can decrease the risk of injuries by helping your joints move through the full range of motion. You may be able to achieve the full range of motion during resistance training, so if time is tight, you can skip stretching.

Daily activities require flexibility, for example, bending down to tie your shoes, reaching overhead to get something from a cupboard, gardening, and getting in and out of a chair or car. Pre-workout dynamic stretching helps you warm up and prevent injuries. Stretching helps improve athletic performance in many, though not all, sports. Post-exercise static stretching feels really good and helps you cool down. I personally recommend it as a way to relax and cool down after a cardio or strength-training workout.

The most common barrier to exercise is lack of time. Wouldn't you like to spend less time working out? The most effective and efficient workouts are high-intensity interval training workouts. These involve short bursts of fast exercise, such as sprinting for up to 30 seconds, with recovery periods of several minutes between bursts. You can complete such a workout in a fraction of the time and get the same or more health benefits compared to a slow and lengthier steady-state aerobic workout such as jogging or walking.

Our brains naturally secrete different neurochemicals. Any neurochemical imbalance can contribute to mild to severe psychological and cognitive problems. Through exercise, we have the power to influence our brain chemistry and help regulate our neurochemicals. For example, exercise increases endorphins, which act as a natural painkiller. Exercise also increases serotonin, which improves our mood, makes us feel more energetic, helps us sleep better, and increases clarity of thought. Exercise, like anti-depressant medications, increases brain-derived neurotropic factor. Regular exercise has been shown to be as effective on mild to moderate depression as antidepressants, without the side effects, and may be an acceptable substitute.

After age 30, the brain starts to lose nerve tissue. Scientists used to believe that each of us is born with a fixed number of neurons that could only decline with age. In recent decades, the theory of neurogenesis—the generation of new neurons in the adult brain—was established. The new neurons are involved in learning, memory, and regulating stress, although the exact relationships are still unclear. Exercise contributes toward the rate of neuron development as well as the survival and functional integration of the new neurons.

Cortisol is another neurochemical. It increases when we're stressed. Chronic stress is harmful. It can result in a high cortisol level, which leads to surplus fuel that ends up being stored as excess belly fat. An overload of cortisol can wreak havoc on the immune system, making us more susceptible to diseases. It can also create a metabolic imbalance, which can lead to diabetes. With exercise, we can burn off stress and reduce cortisol to a productive level. However, excessive exercise, such as frequent high-intensity workouts, can increase cortisol. Too much of a good thing can be bad.

Metabolism decreases by five percent per decade after age 40, which is why we need fewer calories as we age, even if our activity level remains the same, and more so if we become less active. Gender also influences metabolism, with men typically burning more calories at rest than women, because men are naturally more muscular. The more muscular you are, the higher your metabolism. Women tend to shy away from strength training because they're afraid they'll develop massive muscles. That won't happen. Women don't naturally develop big muscles because they have significantly less testosterone than men. Everyone should participate in regular strength training. Muscle burns more calories than fat does, even while at rest. Aerobic exercise and strength training both burn calories, but the latter has a longer-lasting effect on metabolism.

If you want to experience a better quality of life, maybe even increase your life expectancy, I urge you to incorporate cardio, resistance, and flexibility training, along with healthy eating, into your lifestyle. And don't "just do it." Do it like you mean it!

If you're sedentary, you need to have a plan for how you're going to venture into the world of movement. Get the green light from your physician before starting a new exercise program. You can start off with a few minutes of walking several times per week, and progress over time to structured gym workouts or fitness classes, swimming, cycling, tennis, golf, or whatever activities you feel ready to try. The first step is to go from zero to at least doing something at moderate intensity. Once you get into a routine, you need to push yourself—or hire a personal trainer who will push you—to the next level of intensity. I can't tell you how many times I see people pedaling leisurely for a lengthy period of time on a stationary bike while reading a magazine, or walking on a treadmill while watching TV or talking to someone. If you're working at a high level of intensity, you should find it difficult to string together more than a few words. If you can easily chat, read, or watch TV, you're not working hard enough. If you want results, you have to push yourself.

Include more physical activities in your daily life. Don't just think of exercise as a sport or something you do at the gym. Taking the stairs instead of the elevator, parking further away from a building and walking those extra steps, and walking to the corner store rather than driving add up. A few minutes of movement here and there throughout the day can, over the long-term, have a significant impact on your health. Most of the results you'll get from exercise are things you can't see—they happen on the inside. All the incredible health benefits are worth the effort.

Just like a food journal, I recommend keeping an exercise log. While the food journal is meant to be used for a brief period (although those who maintain it for a longer time have more success with weight loss and management), I suggest keeping an exercise log on an ongoing basis. I've kept an exercise log for years. It's a great motivational tool. Here's a sample excerpt from a log. You can record more details if you like, such as listing exactly what exercises you did or your perceived rate of exertion (how difficult you found the workout on a scale of 1 to 10). An activity tracking device is an option. I prefer to keep it simple.

Day, Date, Time	Description of activity, intensity level, duration
Mon., May 1. 7 a.m.	Warm up 10 minutes on stationary bike. Upper-body workout 30 min.
Tue., May 2. 1 p.m.	Run 5 kilometers outdoors in 35 min. Lower-body workout 30 min.
Wed., May 3. 8 a.m.	Walk 30 min. on treadmill at 3.5 miles per hour, increasing incline setting from 1 to 6.
Thu., May 4. 9 a.m. 2 p.m.	60-minute cardio class. 45-minute brisk walk.
Fri., May 5. 8 a.m.	Warm up 10 minutes on rowing machine. Full-body workout for 60 minutes.
Sat., May 6	Did not exercise today.
Sun., May 7. 11 a.m. 3 p.m.	45-minute gentle yoga class. Rollerblading 30 minutes.

When I first started to exercise, I would drag my butt to the gym two or three times per week. You might think that's terrific, but that's actually the recommended *minimum* for strength training. In addition, the recommendation for moderate to vigorous cardiovascular exercise is four to five times per week, or a total of 150 minutes. I wasn't doing anywhere near that. It felt like a real effort going to the gym because my heart wasn't in it. I welcomed any excuse not to go.

It seemed like everyone at the gym had the latest and most fashionable workout clothing. I wore oversized T-shirts emblazoned with geeky software logos and catchphrases. I had one pair of sneakers that were old but had not been used much other than for walking around. I had sweatpants and a pair of baggy shorts. I didn't have any of the cute stuff the other women were wearing.

I did a bit of this and that. I jogged on the treadmill for a few minutes, and then I used a few machines here and there. I was doing something, which was better than nothing. I didn't realize at the time that I didn't have an effective and efficient workout routine. I felt out of my element and hoped that I'd feel more comfortable with time. At least I had a destination every morning, and I wasn't totally embarrassed or ashamed of my body like some people.

Once I began to feel more comfortable exercising and I got into a good routine, I started to work out four to five times per week. Next, I began varying my workouts. If you do the same exercises all the time, your body adapts and you stop seeing results. In addition to doing my own thing on the treadmill and with weights, I finally got the courage to try a fitness class. I hadn't participated in exercise classes in over a decade. I never did enjoy aerobics—and that's okay. You have to keep looking and trying until you find what you enjoy. I tried a class that piqued my interest—cardio skipping. What fun it was. However, during the first couple of weekly classes, I felt a bit faint. I discovered that I definitely needed to eat breakfast before a workout. I also had to drink water before, during, and after the class to replenish my fluids that I lost with all that sweating. Good nutrition and hydration are essential, especially when you're active.

After a few weeks of doing cardio skipping on a weekly basis, I started taking a second class that involved various strength training exercises with dumbbells. At first, I felt like a fish out of water. When I arrived at the class, all the keeners had their mats, color-coded dumbbells, and body bars set up. Luckily, a friend showed me what equipment I needed. After the first class, I was in the know and could fend for myself.

As the weeks and months passed, I noticed more results as my body became leaner and stronger. I started receiving compliments from friends. I wasn't used to the attention of people commenting on my appearance. I rewarded myself with some workout clothes that fit better and I tossed or donated my baggy T-shirts that I'd been using to hide my figure. Like an onion, I began to peel back the exterior layers and reveal my slowly-changing body.

A friend I hadn't seen in a while gave me a thumbs up as he drove by and shouted, "You look so fit!"

Another friend greeted me with "Hi Skinny!"

Some people at the gym asked me how I lost weight. I was slim (but not necessarily fit) until I was in my late thirties, yet I never got those kinds of compliments or requests for advice back then. I realized that many people were now impressed with my notable progress. Not only had I slimmed down, but I looked fit.

When I hired Gina to show me the correct way to use the equipment and to set up a workout routine, I felt a bit intimidated. She was a few years older than me; however, she was in great physical shape. Surprisingly, after a few sessions, I felt that I no longer needed a trainer. I'd become intrinsically motivated! How did I know that? I was keen to learn and work out on my own. I scoured the Internet and fitness magazines to select interesting and more advanced exercises that kept me challenged. Soon, I was even demonstrating new exercises for my friends so they could try them. I would never have predicted that I'd come to such a point where I actually enjoyed working out hard and sweating.

⚜

One day, I nearly sustained serious injury while attempting a risky exercise. I'd seen one of the trainers, Lynne, doing handstand push-ups against a wall in the gym. Lynne is the same age as me. At that time, we were in our mid-forties. Everyone who witnessed Lynne doing this freakishly difficult exercise was impressed. She asked me to try a handstand push-up and offered to spot me, but I knew I couldn't do it and didn't want to embarrass myself. I decided to try the exercise in the privacy of my home where I thought I could perfect it.

The most I could do was a headstand up against my bedroom wall. I couldn't lift myself up onto my hands. Never in my life have I done a handstand. It just looked so cool and I wanted to give it a try. I slipped and fell, twisting my neck as I hit the floor. I lay there momentarily, afraid to move. I thought I might have paralyzed myself! After a few minutes, I dared to try to get up off of the floor. Fortunately, I could. My hand was tingling. I must have slightly injured a nerve. I was sore and stiff for days. I never tried that again.

My advice to you is don't go overboard. Enthusiasm is a good thing, and I urge everyone to push themselves; however, if you take on too many activities, push yourself too hard, or forget to make safety a priority, you become susceptible to injuries as well as psychological burnout. Exercise attrition is high for beginners, especially those who do too much, too quickly.

⚜

I knew I had arrived at a new turning point in my transformation when I was upset that the gym would be closed on certain days, or if

I had an appointment that interfered with my workout schedule. Just months prior, I had embraced any opportunity *not* to go to the gym. The repairman is coming to the house so I can't go to the gym. Jesse and Joshua have no school today so I can't go to the gym. The new me had no time for excuses! I'd go to the gym after my appointment. I'd bring the boys with me to the gym and have them play or read in a safe area while I worked out. The new me *wanted* to exercise.

I was proud of myself. I was now exercising five mornings per week and I loved it. Some seven or eight months had passed since I made up my mind to get fit. In that time, I'd lost nearly 20 pounds and I went from a size 11/12 to a size 8. I hadn't worn an 8 in over a decade. I had much better muscle tone all around. My pants were literally falling off me. My waist and tummy were much smaller now. I wanted to wear a dress that I'd bought just months prior, and when I tried it on, I felt like I was swimming in it. It was much too loose at the waist. At the time I'd bought it, I thought it was cute and attractive; now, I found it to be frumpy. I wanted a shorter dress that hugged my new figure.

Another indication that I was evolving came when Allan and I were planning a summer vacation. The boys would be at sleep-away camp, just the opportunity for Allan and me to go on a romantic getaway. Previously, we'd considered going to a spa for some rest and relaxation; however, I was now craving action. I convinced Allan that we needed a trip that combined relaxation and adventure. I got online and googled "adventure vacations." I found something that sounded exciting: heli-hiking. This four-day trip would take place in British Columbia. Each day, guests would be flown in a helicopter to a location in the mountains above the tree line. We would hike through scenic, unspoiled landscapes, and return to the lodge for gourmet dining, hot tubbing, and stretching classes. It sounded like a dream!

Over time, my exercise regimen became more comprehensive, with increasingly challenging strength training and cardiovascular exercise, and stretching to improve my flexibility. Who knew what was next on the horizon? Perhaps yoga. Okay, I wasn't quite ready for yoga just yet. Or was I?

Gloria Schwartz

Personal Best Exercises

o Select some days and times that you can devote to exercise each week and figure out how to arrange your schedule so you can stick to your plan.

o List three new types of physical activities that you're willing to try several times in order to discover what you enjoy.

o Find out everything you need to know to prepare for your new activities; for example, where and when you can participate in them, whether you need to register, what gear you need to buy or borrow, and how much time you'll need for the activity including travel time and showering/changing.

Did you know?

• It's advisable to warm up for five to ten minutes before you exercise. This will reduce your risk of injury.

• Strength training isn't just for bodybuilders. It improves functional fitness in people of all ages. It increases bone density and decreases the risk of fractures in post-menopausal women. Even people in their 90s can significantly increase their muscle mass and mobility with regular strength training.

• It's normal to experience muscular soreness for up to 48 hours following exercise. You should allow your muscles to rest and recover for 48 hours between workouts so muscle fibers can repair, which is how your muscles get bigger and stronger. It's not normal to experience pain during or after exercise.

• Exercise is not a license to eat with wild abandon. Rewarding yourself with a big meal or treats can lead to weight gain. It's easy to hoover a 250-calorie chocolate bar in a few minutes, but it can take approximately 30 minutes of exercise to burn off those calories.

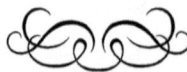

6 SUPPORT

The brain is the hardest part of the body to train.

A support system is an important part of the blueprint. If you don't have support from the people around you, you may feel alienated, or pressured to engage in counterproductive behaviors. Your friends and family do not have to necessarily live the life you are now living; but it's best if they're supportive of your endeavors. They must respect your philosophy. This can be tough. Some friends and family members may overtly—or even worse, covertly—attempt to sabotage you. Subconsciously, they may not want you to change or to succeed. They'd never admit it, but they may be jealous that you're losing weight and getting fit. Some clients have confided in me that they suspect that their husbands don't want them to lose weight. Why? One reason may be that the husbands are worried that their wives will get more attention from other men. Some saboteurs may simply prefer the familiar person they used to know—not the new, emerging one who opts out of an all-you-can-eat pizza and wings night.

As you start changing, you'll understand that it's more comfortable for other people to deal with the status quo than with your changes. Change requires introspection and effort. As you work on self-improvement, you may inadvertently shine a spotlight on areas where your friends or family members could use improvement. This can be emotionally painful for them to deal with. They may feel threatened. It's easier for them if you don't change because then they don't have to confront their own feelings and shortcomings.

Like a reformed drug addict who is forced to walk away from

her set of druggie friends, if you're going to have long-term success with your new lifestyle, you need to immerse yourself in a new environment that provides a culture of health and positivity. That means surrounding yourself with like-minded people who live a healthy lifestyle and understand your new direction. If you continue to hang around with enablers, overeaters, and people who don't care about their health and wellness, it will be harder for you to continue making positive choices. If you dine with old cronies who regularly eat fattening, super-sized snacks and meals, then you run the risk of reverting to your old habits. People who dine with overeaters tend to overeat as well. Environmental cues are a major cause of relapse.

Even a simple dinner party at someone's home can trigger old habits. I've been served meals laden with fat and salt, such as pasta in creamy sauces, fatty cuts of meat in gravy, and salads smothered in heavy dressing. The worst type of experience for me is when a well-intentioned hostess serves me, rather than letting me choose what I want. I've been handed plates piled high with enough food to feed my whole family! The host or hostess thinks they're being generous. We've been raised to equate food with love, but that's an attempt to kill me with kindness! Looking at a plate like that makes me uncomfortable. It's overwhelming. I much prefer eating at the homes of the more health-conscious, where the food is typically healthy, I can select what I want and take right-sized portions, and I don't end up wasting unwanted food or getting indigestion.

If you have extreme willpower and self-discipline, then continue associating with negative influences. The truth is, if you had extreme willpower, you probably wouldn't be reading this book and looking for help. Why put yourself at an increased risk of failure? Just as you must make strategic decisions about food and exercise, so too must you make strategic decisions about the people you spend time with and how you spend that time. Friends and family should be part of the solution, not part of the problem.

You deserve better than saboteurs and naysayers. This is not to say that you must abandon your friends and family if they are not supportive or if they lead a different lifestyle. That's not always realistic, nor is it what you necessarily want, especially because those relationships likely add value in other ways. Plus, you can't control the world around you. Just because you're changing, that doesn't mean everyone else has to change in order to accommodate you. A more practical strategy is to work on internal change by consciously deciding who you will allow to influence you and how you'll cope with negative influences.

One way to deal with negative influences is to carefully consider the sorts of activities you'll participate in with these people. Perhaps meet them for tea rather than for dinner. Suggest meeting up for a walk and make sure you bypass the donut shop. You never know who will be receptive to your suggestions. If you're invited to someone's home and you know, based on experience, that the food will not suit you, ask the host if you can bring your own meal, or offer to bring a couple of dishes for everyone so that you'll have some healthy options.

If you'll be attending a social event that revolves around food, as do many events, plan and rehearse before you go. Think about how you'll respond when faced with temptations. If you're going to have an indulgence, make it a conscious one that you've thought through.

What should you do if friends repeatedly attempt to dissuade you from your goals by planting seeds of doubt in your mind about your abilities, by putting you down in other ways, or by insisting you eat things that aren't in your plan? True friends should not make you feel bad about yourself. True friends should be supportive and have your best interest at heart. Make your expectations clear to them. Make sure you stay away from a toxic environment.

Before I began my journey, I thought that if I hung out with people who weighed more and ate more than me, then I would look great in comparison. That was my not-so-brilliant theory of relativity. Now I know that was a mistake. Becoming a better me is not about stroking my ego or enjoying a moment of schadenfreude. It's not about looking or feeling better than anyone else. It's about being a better me than my former self. It's about reaching for the stars and working for what I truly desire.

Once I started losing weight and feeling better about myself, and once I got to know some of the fit people at the gym, I started to feel as though I wanted to hang out with some of them. Perhaps I could learn from their example. Now that I was on the right track, I felt as though I had something in common with the fit set. Some of the trainers invited me to social get-togethers and we became friendly.

My new acquaintances understood what I wanted for myself. They appreciated the efforts I was making to improve my fitness and health. Hanging out with them helped me stay on the right path, not only because they modelled positive lifestyle behaviors, but because I would have felt ashamed exhibiting poor eating habits in front of them. With my old buddies, there was no shame in eating greasy food or relying on eating as our core activity. The more I observed others modeling healthy behaviors, the more I became convinced that I could do the same without feeling deprived.

The "humiliation factor" is a term I use to describe a type of negative reinforcer that has the potential to deliver positive results. The humiliation factor plays a big role when it comes to eating and exercising. In my case, when I first got started on the road to self-improvement, I had to be at the gym if I was going to exercise properly. Sure, I'd bought instructional DVDs and assorted exercise equipment over the years, but until I saw the light, I was not really motivated to push myself, especially when I tried to work out at home on my own. If I started following an exercise DVD in the privacy of my home, I'd stop as soon as a droplet of sweat excreted from my forehead, if the phone rang, if my toe hurt, if I had a hunger pang, or if I realized it was Arbor Day and I had to go plant a tree. Any excuse to stop and I latched onto it.

At the gym, I was motivated by the humiliation factor. I didn't stop exercising as a result of feeling humiliated; rather, I exercised longer and with greater intensity in order to *prevent* feelings of humiliation. People were watching me. No, I'm not a paranoid schizophrenic. They weren't directly observing me and taking notes, but they could see what I was up to, just as I noticed what they were doing. I was ashamed to stop after one push-up or two sit-ups. If everyone else in a fitness class could do the moves, why not me? Sometimes I couldn't keep up with the instructor or other participants, but I still kept going at my own pace. I didn't stop and sit down as I would have done at home where no one could see me give up. That would have been embarrassing. Eventually, my shame-avoidance was replaced with pride. I became proud of my new physical abilities and felt motivated to try harder, whether I was in the company of others or alone.

As for eating, the humiliation factor played a big role, too. Many of us are secret eaters, aren't we? How many times have you had company over for dinner or a party and you just nibbled at the food, but then after everyone left, you polished off the leftovers? I confess I've done that time and again. In front of people, I might just eat a few chips, but when the party's over and that half bag is calling my name, my head ploughs straight into it like a horse at a trough. If a tree falls in the forest and no one is there to hear it, does it make a sound? There's no humiliation if no one can see what you're doing— or is there? When I took ownership of my actions and accepted that I have the power to make intelligent decisions about what I eat, I learned to put away the leftovers rather than binge on them. No guilt. No shame.

ɩɩ

One thing I discovered, which surprised me, is that even people who are super fit and healthy actually enjoy eating some of the foods that I do. I used to think that very slim and fit people, especially those who work in the fitness industry, eat like birds. Not true. Skinny people may under eat, but healthy, fit, active people eat well. They fuel their bodies. And they know how to enjoy good food in moderation. I know that now because I'm one of those fit people. But back then I realized, by associating myself with some positive role models, that you can still enjoy a variety of delicious foods and a treat on occasion, without guilt. Why no guilt? Because if your overall lifestyle is a healthy one, if you're exercising regularly, participating in physical activities, and eating healthily day to day, then there's no guilt or shame in treating yourself.

I'm not a proponent of total deprivation. I recommend the 80/20 rule of thumb. Treat your body well at least 80 percent of the time, and relax and enjoy yourself up to 20 percent of the time.

ɩɩ

One of the people who encouraged me early on in my journey was Sandy, a woman whom I usually saw five times a week when we picked our sons up from school. We'd chat in the parking lot.

"What did you eat today?" Sandy would ask jokingly. I'd confess all my food sins to her and she'd confess hers to me. This exercise helped me become more accountable for my eating at a time when I was still frequenting fast-food restaurants. When I'd confess my daily sins to my friend by articulating what I'd indulged in that day, I started becoming more self-aware and slowly revised my choices. Again, the humiliation factor took hold. I laughed, but I was a bit embarrassed about some of the horrible things I admitted to her that I'd eaten, so I started eating a little less horribly. We consoled each other when we had bad eating days, and we gave each other positive feedback and compliments on good days. Everyone can benefit from such a confidant. Do you have someone like that in your life who is non-judgmental?

❧❧

Resistance you get from family or friends may leave you feeling aggravated or emotionally drained. You may find you're spending precious time trying to change their attitude instead of spending that time on bettering yourself. Make the tough decisions—keep trying to get them to be supportive, or move on. I suggest that you focus on what is within your control. Focus on what you need and go after it.

One evening, Allan said he had to run to the convenience store to pick up some snacks that we could eat later that evening during the season finale of our favorite TV show. I told him that we had plenty of snacks at home—grapes, apples, cheese, and water. He felt that I was spoiling his fun. He said if I didn't want to eat chips or whatever he'd buy, I didn't have to. I got mad. If I were an alcoholic, would he bring alcohol home and expect me to have enough willpower to resist the temptation while he drank it in front of me? I accused him of trying to sabotage my efforts and I told him if he bought chips, he'd better eat them in the car. He looked at me like a deer in the headlights, and then he decided to have some fruit instead. My aim was not to make him eat fruit (okay, maybe it was). I just didn't want those darn chips in my face when I'd been trying so hard to change bad habits. Sometimes people are just not attuned to your needs and you must make your expectations clear.

In the past, if I couldn't find someone to do an activity with me, I wouldn't do it on my own. For example, I found jogging boring by myself. Same for going to the gym. Maybe that's because I was trying to look at physical activities as purely social—I really wasn't interested in the exercise aspect. So if I didn't have a buddy, I didn't do it. I've come to realize that it's up to me to do things, with or without someone. As a matter of fact, I now prefer the independence of just doing things on my own, such as going to the gym without having to expend energy trying to convince or coordinate friends to join me. I go ahead on my own and if I feel like doing some socializing, I chat a bit with some people at the gym or wherever I happen to be. It's a good way to meet new people and it enables me to be free to do as I please. I can no longer fool myself into believing that I can't work out because so-and-so isn't available to go with me. I'm a big girl. I'm responsible for myself and what I do. So I just do it.

When it comes to support, we must be our own best friend. Sadly, many of us have been our own worst enemy for so long that we aren't even cognizant of our self-defeating thoughts and actions.

Sometimes we deny our true value as human beings and we only see weaknesses within ourselves. We dissect every aspect of who we are and put ourselves down. This negativity can pertain to anything from physical attributes to behaviors and personality traits. Sadly, I often encounter people who live in self-judgment mode. When I compliment female friends on how slim or fit they look, instead of a thank-you or acknowledgement, I'm typically received with unrealistic, negative self-perceptions such as, "But my thighs look huge," or "If only my stomach didn't stick out so much."

Many years ago I didn't know how to respond when I received compliments. I would feel a bit embarrassed or uncomfortable. I often employed self-deprecating humor. At the time, I talked to a friend about my issue and she gave me some simple but effective advice. She suggested that I smile and say, "Why thank you!" That was wonderful advice because it didn't require me to directly address or debate a compliment; but it did mean that I was accepting it whether or not I agreed with it. And once I learned to accept a compliment without expressing doubt, I actually started to believe in the positives and think less about my self-doubts. It's sort of like the idea that if you intentionally smile or laugh for no particular reason, you'll start to feel happier. This is due to cognitive dissonance. Our brains needs to close the gap between that which we believe and that which we do. If we do something often enough that is inconsistent with our thoughts, our brains will make us begin to think in new ways to better align our thoughts with our actions. If we accept compliments rather than look for evidence to dispel them, we'll start to believe them. Accepting compliments will then become more natural and psychologically comfortable for us.

I've said it before and I'll say it again: The brain is the hardest part of the body to train. We must train our brains to do away with self-defeating thoughts. Accept compliments at face value rather than deflect or deconstruct them. Think of a compliment as a reward for your efforts. If we fail to see our own shining light, let others point it out to us. From there, our self-esteem will flourish.

In 2013, I began giving motivational talks. At my very first talk, I asked the attendees—who all happened to be female—to write one thing they wished they could change about themselves. I also asked them to write one thing they most liked about themselves. One of the women asked me to clarify whether I meant something physical or non-physical. I told her that whatever she wanted to write was fine. When all the women had put down their pens, I asked for volunteers to read aloud what they wished they could change about themselves. Almost everyone's hand shot up. Answers were called out: "my big thighs," "my flabby stomach," and "my jiggly upper arms." When I asked for volunteers to read aloud what they most liked about themselves, the room fell silent. I eventually convinced a few women to volunteer what they liked about themselves: "my smile" and "my ears." Many of these educated and accomplished women—like so many women—seemed to have a poor self-image when it came to their bodies.

Most people want to change something about themselves. We tend to compare ourselves to others. There are times when it's useful to do so; but it can be a slippery slope. There will always be someone better looking, slimmer, fitter, funnier, more artistic, wealthier, or whatever. If we compare ourselves to others, we may become disappointed that we cannot be like this person or that person.

Similarly, there will always be someone less fit, someone who runs more slowly, someone with less talent, and so on. If we compare ourselves to them, it might stroke our egos, but we may not be motivated to achieve our full potential. We may become complacent and believe that we are good enough. Each of us has to figure out when we are content with being good enough at something, and when we are prepared to push ourselves beyond mediocrity. We need to accept ourselves and appreciate ourselves, but we also must push ourselves to be able to achieve our personal best.

Standing in line behind a morbidly obese person at the chip wagon might make you think that you look really good, and that you can eat whatever you want. In reality, you might be overweight to a lesser degree and need to watch what you consume. People who socialize a lot with heavy people tend to underestimate how overweight they themselves are. They compare themselves to their social counterparts and form an incorrect mental model of what "normal" looks like.

Even if you're not overweight, why eat that garbage? Prevention is the key to good health, and that involves making intelligent choices. Damage to our bodies begins at the vascular and cellular level long before symptoms appear or before diagnosis, in most cases, is even possible. So don't compare yourself to others when making choices for yourself. Eat for health, no matter what you look like. When you train your brain, you'll realize that healthy eating is pleasurable.

We need to find the sweet spot. The best way to do that is to leverage others who display positive behaviors. Those people can be our allies, our role models, and our mentors. We can learn better skills and habits from them. We need to also recognize that those people have their own insecurities and weak points. It's counterproductive to want to be like someone else in any way, if the comparison causes us to diminish our own sense of self-worth or to be constantly self-critical.

❧❧❧

No one is perfect. What is good, bad, beautiful, or ugly is an individual assessment often influenced by societal values. What may be considered beautiful now may be out of fashion next month.

We can achieve our full potential if we focus on being the best that we can be. To do that, it's necessary to have a realistic view of ourselves, to be introspective, and to set increasingly challenging but achievable goals. We must look at where we are today, how far we have come, and where we want to be tomorrow. When clients or friends ask me for advice, they sometimes respond to my suggestions with a knee-jerk reaction of excuses. That makes me think, "How's that been working for you?" If what you've been doing (or not doing) isn't working for you, then take the advice of someone who knows! If you can't objectively analyze your behavioral and thought patterns, let an expert assist you.

If you don't know where you want to be, how will you get there? Once you assess yourself and define your goals, you can follow the path necessary for achievement. Sure, some things just happen through luck or because they are meant to be. You might land a job or meet your life partner via a chance encounter. However, you're more likely to achieve your goals if you plan them and work towards them. Look at both the big picture and the details of your physical, emotional, and spiritual self in the past, present, and future. You need to focus on what went well in the past, what didn't go so well, areas for improvement, and what you could have done differently. There's no use beating yourself up for past failures. Learn from the past. Use your experiences as tools. Apply what you learn so that you can shape your thoughts and behaviors and change in ways that you desire. This constant process of reviewing, learning, and applying knowledge will propel you towards where you are going, and beyond!

When I first started attending fitness classes, I found them tough. That was to be expected since I was not in great condition. Also, a good class is supposed to provide a challenge. If it's easy, what's the point? The instructors and fellow participants were supportive. That really encouraged me. Sometimes, all we need is a positive stroke such as a high-five or to hear someone tell us, "Good job!"

After I held to my commitment for many months, I started to find those same classes were not all that challenging anymore. I needed something new that would push me more, now that I was in better physical and mental shape. The instructor who was teaching cardio kickboxing suggested that I come to his karate school so I could try a kickboxing class where you get to hit targets rather than hitting the air. By hitting a target, the resistance would work the muscles throughout my body much better. I didn't really care about the benefit as much as the fun I thought it would be. I tried out the class. The instructor paired me up with another woman who happened to be half my age and about twice my weight. I was a bit intimidated at first. I thought she was going to kill me! I asked her not to hurt me. I said a little prayer. Fortunately, we did not make contact with one another in this class. We took turns holding a punching bag and performed punching and kicking combos on it. I really found the class exhilarating and empowering. I never sweated so much in one hour. What? I now enjoyed working up a sweat? This was not princess-style exercise. This was tough, tough, tough! My arms were aching by the end of the class. My partner high-fived me. I felt like Rocky.

In order to stay motivated and continue to improve yourself, you need to find new challenges and set increasingly challenging goals for yourself. You need to find something you love. You need to be inspired. The best way to find that is to try different things. Maybe kickboxing is not for you, but unless you try a few different activities, you won't know. I'd found my next level of energy and drive and I was going to apply it to push the limits and see where I could go.

After many months of hard work and a progression of incremental successes that eventually snowballed into tangible achievement, I knew I'd arrived when I received an email from Lynne, the trainer. In what turned out to be a prophetic email, she wrote:

> "You're my new inspiration at the gym to keep challenging myself and my clients with new and interesting workouts. You've done a great job training yourself Gloria and the results show! Maybe you have a future as a personal trainer?"

I was floored by the email. It really touched me. This woman, who'd been entrenched in a healthy lifestyle all of her life, found *me* to be an inspiration. Those few words had so much power. Those words were like the nectar of the gods. I drank them in. I felt that someone I looked up to was acknowledging me. Those words

71

psychologically catapulted me to the next level. With those words, I knew I was finally ready to challenge myself even more. I now believed that I could accomplish any fitness goal—anything at all—if I put my mind to it.

Any remaining vestiges of self-doubt vanished. I suddenly understood that whatever direction I would go in, I would somehow take others along for the ride with me. I was no longer just trying to lose a few more inches or become a bit more muscular. Instead, I was ready to head down a path that included more self-awareness and introspection. I wanted to better understand what was important to me and to my happiness at this stage of my life and I wanted others to feel the same exhilaration. I was ready to open my mind to experiences that went beyond being fit, looking good, or getting healthier. Now I was ready to consider more abstract ways of thinking. Perhaps meditation or some other way to become more enlightened. When I told Allan that I wanted to attend a meditation class, he looked at me funny. I didn't care if he thought I was getting flakey. I felt self-assured and I was moving forward.

I was now in a stage of mental preparedness that surprised me. One day, while running, I started hearing a song in my head that became my running mantra.

"This train is bound for glory, this train. This train is bound for glory, this train." I realized the lyrics were from a pre-Civil War emancipation spiritual. Was I subconsciously freeing myself from my self-imposed manacles of doubt? Like a broken record, the lyrics played over and over in my head as I ran, giving me the focus and will to keep going.

The new me wanted to expand my horizons. The new me wanted to show others what was possible. I was ready. Look out world. Here I come!

By now, I'd achieved my weight loss goals, including revised ones. I'd become lean and fit. I'd lost several dress sizes. I'd adopted a new, healthier lifestyle that included not just pure exercise, but fun physical activities. I'd modified my eating habits over time and I was now on the right track. I was no longer a slave to temptations and not as easily swayed by the negative influences of others. I'd surrounded myself with more positive influences and role models who inspired me to challenge myself. I'd learned to accept my imperfections and go forward. I'd learned to graciously accept compliments and pat myself on the back. I'd come so far. I felt like I was at a juncture and I thought, "Now what?"

I had an epiphany. I realized that long-term personal success would not be enough. I decided I wanted to help other people like me get motivated. That's why I wrote this book. Every day I see people who are just like I was not long ago. I hope that by sharing my experiences, my knowledge, and my passion, I can inspire you.

Although it's now been years since the beginning of my journey, I still continue to learn and grow. I have a lifetime—a lifetime of working at maintaining my commitment to myself.

At times, I feel as though my previous ways were an addiction that are currently lying dormant somewhere in me, waiting to surface if I let down my guard. It would be all too easy to stop exercising and revert to eating poorly. I still feel temptations at times and I have to convince myself to eat this and not that. I don't win every battle. When I make a poor choice, I forgive myself and get back on the right path. It gets easier with time to combat my demons, but I have to keep working at it. This admission is for you, to let you know that whatever struggles you encounter, you're not alone. No one said it would be easy. The beauty of success is the hard work we put into achieving it.

The journey never really ends. When the student becomes the teacher—that is, a role model and an inspiration for others—then the next phase of the journey begins. It's amazing how a bit of inspiration and a lot of perspiration can lead to incredible results.

Personal Best Exercises

○ Identify someone you currently know who is a good role model for fitness and healthy living. How does that person inspire you? Ask that person if he or she is willing to be your mentor.

○ Describe a failure you had at some point with improving your fitness or eating habits. How can you use this experience as a learning opportunity?

○ List three things about yourself that you like and explain why. They can be physical attributes, personality traits, or behaviors.

Did you know?

• Getting your family to support and encourage your goals may require you to communicate what it is *specifically* that you'd like them to do. For example, if they continue eating junk food, ask them not to bring it into the house, or to eat it in another room and not in front of you. You may want to clarify and confirm your needs to ensure all parties understand and agree to the new "rules."

• Although it helps to have friends and family onboard, it's not essential to your success. It's really up to you to learn to cope and make sound decisions that support your goals and plans.

• An organized support group can be beneficial for those who are comfortable discussing their progress with like-minded people in a non-threatening environment.

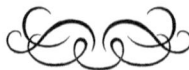

7 MAINTENANCE

Persist and persevere.

Long-term maintenance doesn't just happen on its own. You need to factor it into your blueprint. Perhaps the two biggest obstacles that stand between you and success are: 1- finding the motivation to get started, and 2- maintaining that motivation long term in order to preserve the fruits of your labor and continue to improve on them.

Many people set goals and achieve them, but for one reason or another they end up back at square one. For example, they lose a certain amount of weight, but they eventually gain it back and then some. You can maintain what you've accomplished and even continue to improve in the long term, if you set both short- and long-term goals. You must also make a personal commitment to stick with fitness and intelligent eating habits as a lifestyle, rather than seeking a quick fix and a short-term solution.

How do you know when you've achieved your current goals and are ready for maintenance mode? In the first place, you had to have set some goals. If, for example, your goal was to get down to a certain weight, then it's pretty obvious when you've achieved your goal. But is weight really the ultimate measure of success? Even a slender person can be unfit or unhealthy. I recommend that you focus on fitness and health, rather than purely on the numbers on the scale.

As for my own progress, I began to consider what I needed to do to maintain my weight, my level of fitness, and my improved health indicators.

Gloria Schwartz

After all those months of hard work, I asked myself what I could do to keep up my level of activity, knowing that I had a big obstacle in my path. I'd be spending most of the summer at my cottage, away from the city, with no gym in the vicinity.

I made a plan. I bought an exercise ball and some dumbbells for the cottage, and I brought my kickboxing DVD and boxing gloves from home so I could do some exercises. I even brought my boxing bag that I'd received as a Mother's Day gift a few years earlier and which had been gathering dust in my basement closet.

My plan would also include kayaking and lots of running on hilly country roads. I set a target for myself to run at least 200 kilometers over the next two months, roughly 25 kilometers per week. That target turned out to be a bit too ambitious, but it did give me something to strive for.

I prepared a chart to log my activities. I would be fully responsible for my own workouts, with no fitness professionals in close proximity to give me helpful tips or positive strokes. This would be a big psychological test for me. Would I be able to remain active on a daily basis or would I revert to my lethargic ways? While I was a bit concerned, I felt deep down that I could keep up the efforts. I could be stronger and leaner or I could return to my old, out-of-shape self. My eye was on the prize and I was not going to lose sight of it.

❧

Just before I left the city for my summer at the cottage, my former trainer Gina invited me to her house for a pool party. It sounded like fun until I realized that some of my remaining insecurities about my body would be magnified. How could I wear my new itsy-bitsy bikini in front of Gina and Lynne—both trainers with awesome figures? Maybe I should wear board shorts that go down to my knees, I thought to myself, or a muumuu.

When I really thought about it, I knew I looked pretty good, especially when compared to my former self just months ago. I reminded myself that I must not compare myself to anyone else. I hoped everyone would be supportive and that my only true critic would be me. I was my best friend, but at times, my worst enemy. Off to the pool party went this warrior; after all, warriors have no fear and they surely don't hesitate to wear a bikini. The party turned out to be a lot of fun and I felt very comfortable wearing my bikini.

⚜

That July and August, I stuck to my plan of taking care of myself, maintaining my weight and level of activity, and watching what I ate. I did eat a bit of junk food, but I kept it to a minimum compared to how I ate the previous summer. For example, I'd have two or three cookies instead of a dozen, or a few crackers and cheese instead of half a box of crackers. I kept chips and ice cream to a real minimum, just a few times over the course of the summer. I was proud of how far I'd come. Some people might think it's terrible to include junk food when claiming to be living a healthy lifestyle, but I knew that's what worked for me. Going off of all junk food cold turkey would have turned me into a stressed-out, crazy woman and I would have given up.

2008 would become my summer of love—of loving and taking care of myself without outside help, without access to a professional gym, and without like-minded people nearby to encourage me. The previous summer, the old me would sit on the dock at the lake and eat chips. Now the new me laid out a towel on the dock and did push-ups, sit-ups, planks, stretching, and meditation. The new me had the confidence to run on the hilly unpaved roads around the cottage and work towards my goals.

I read some magazines that featured success stories and before-and-after photos. A light bulb went off in my head. I asked Allan to take a front, side, and rear photo of me in my new bikini, to use as my benchmark. I'd come a long way since a year before when I was flabby and unfit; but I still wanted to improve myself, and these photos would allow me to see the progress I anticipated I'd make in the next few months. I cringed when I saw my side photo—my tummy still stuck out; however, I knew I was in much better shape now than I'd been in several years.

I gleaned some useful tips from magazines, including working on my positive self-talk and affirmations. I wrote "I am a warrior" on a piece of paper and stuck it on the bathroom mirror. Every day when I saw that quote, I felt ready to tackle the hills on my run and ready to try new and more challenging activities. Years later, that paper is still there, yellowed and faded. It continues to inspire me.

After a couple of tries, I was able to run over four kilometers to the end of the road, panting as I pushed my way up each hill, and silently revelling as I stormed down each hill. I even recruited my neighbor Marie to join me whenever she was at her cottage. With her as my running buddy, the time seemed to fly. It was rewarding to see her sense of accomplishment after she finished her first run with me. She hadn't thought she could run that far on such hilly roads. When we saw the mailboxes around the bend, knowing that we were almost there, we both felt elated.

The summer was turning out great. I began to think of new ways to vary my workouts and help others. I read about fartleks, which I thought were emergency bathroom stops that I had to do on occasion in the woods when nature called. I learned that fartleks are running workouts that entail quick, short spurts of speed mixed with longer, slower-paced runs. I read sports psychology and fitness motivation university textbooks, as I became increasingly interested in understanding what drives ordinary people like me to convert to a fitness philosophy. Plenty of research lay ahead, as it was just early July, but I knew in my heart that I was on a path of learning that would lead to something good.

Meanwhile, I achieved a goal that I had set for myself a few weeks prior, a goal that I had planned on achieving before the end of summer. This was the goal to run to the mailboxes at the end of the road and all the way back without stopping once. The route had several long and steep inclines. On July 10, I just told myself, "Today's the day" and I set out on my own with the intention of going for it with every bit of energy I had in me.

At about the 6 kilometer mark, as I reached the foot of the hill I nicknamed "Diablo" because of how steep and tough it was, I thought I wouldn't make it. Just as I felt like giving up, as I was half way up Diablo, panting, my quads burning, I repeated my mantra in my head, "This train is bound for glory" and I kept going. It was the toughest run I ever did. When I got to the top of Diablo, I knew I'd be able to finish the last couple of kilometers. There were still a few hills ahead but they were not as difficult.

I noticed the sound of my running shoes as they hit the gravel road with each step, my cadence like a metronome. I thought how wonderful it would be to have a recording of the sound of my footsteps as I ran in the mental zone with every ounce of energy, a hypnotic rhythm that would remind me of this momentous day. When I got to the end of my run, I was filled with emotion, a real sense of accomplishment and euphoria. I had done something that months ago would have seemed like an impossible dream, beyond my reach. Now it was complete. Now I was ready to start thinking of my next goal.

ɩɣ

Not only was I active most of the summer, but sometimes I even ran when it rained. And I ran when the bugs were out in full force. I bought a bug net to wear over my head. I looked like a beekeeper. I persisted, running with horse flies and other annoying, hungry insects swarming around me. I thought I was safe with my bug net, but I soon discovered that they found other places to bite me. That summer, I had at least 50 insect bites on my back at any given time. I spent many nights scratching endlessly. But I felt tough. I felt unstoppable!

ɩɣ

For me, maintenance mode took on a whole new meaning. I came to realize that I did not want to "maintain" a particular status quo. I didn't want to stop improving.

I'm not talking about weight. Don't get me wrong. Weight obsession is unhealthy. Nope, that wasn't my issue. While I truly recognized how far I'd come, I was always looking ahead to see what I could dream of next. I wanted to set the bar a little higher each time. How could I continue to challenge myself mentally and physically so that I could truly feel like the warrior that I strived to be?

ɩɣ

One day in early August, I managed to do one full chin-up on the horizontal bar on our swing set. I had tried unsuccessfully for so long that I thought it was a fluke. I tried again the next day to see if I could replicate it. Voila! I did it. Months of persistence had paid off. I

79

could finally pull up my full body weight from extended arms to chin height. I felt like a champion. This was my proof that one can achieve so much when one makes a commitment.

⚜

On some days when the rain was heavy and I needed a change of scenery, I drove an hour to the city and went to the gym. One day, I noticed a woman who seemed to be reluctantly exercising under Lynne's guidance. The woman asked me how I was so motivated to put in so much effort. I didn't have an answer for her because I could have talked for hours about finding my inner warrior. I observed her as Lynne coaxed and cajoled her into doing another rep of a chest press with light dumbbells. I could see at a glance that this woman was going through the motions. While a trainer is there to help motivate the client, the reality is that paying someone to coach you will only yield results if you are truly sold on the idea and willing to put in the effort. I wanted to scream at the woman, "Do it like you mean it!" but luckily my filter was turned on and I kept my thoughts to myself. If only this woman could understand how good it feels to put in a consistent effort and see results. I wished at that moment that I could help her see the light. At that time, I was not a personal trainer, but something inside of me wanted to help her. That woman needed so much more than someone to show her proper exercise techniques; she needed a motivational coach to speak the truth, not pamper her. It was apparent to me that she was not yet in the right stage of mental readiness. Yes, she was in the Action stage. She was going through the motions, but she wasn't fully engaged. She didn't believe in herself so she couldn't see the possibilities. She wasn't inspired to turn inspiration into meaningful action—even though between Lynne and myself she had sources of inspiration right in front of her eyes. I've seen many people just like that woman. I used to be one of them.

⚜

If you open your eyes and your mind and make yourself receptive, you'll find sources of inspiration all around you. Observing and learning from those sources can have a powerfully motivating effect. That motivation makes long-term maintenance possible.

If you're lucky, you may meet a few people in your lifetime who inspire and motivate you in unexpected ways when you least expect it and most need it. Take, for example, Bette.

I met Bette on a mountain top, literally. Allan and I were on the heli-hiking vacation we'd planned. Each day, we and a small group of other hikers were flown in a helicopter from our lodge and dropped off with a guide in a remote location in the Columbian mountains of British Columbia. The thrill of flying in a helicopter was surpassed by the awe-inspiring landscapes that ranged from rocky terrain as high and wide as the eye can see, to meadows covered in Red Paintbrush and other brightly-hued wildflowers, to ice fields and ice caves, to emerald lakes. During this adventure, I realized how much I had missed out on over the years when I was not in a state of mind to try physically-demanding vacations. We hiked where few people get to go, making ascents where the only occasional path was created by goats. We descended into valleys that were created 600 million years ago.

Bette was the oldest person in our group, but I didn't know her age. We chatted as we hiked. She was full of energy. She not only kept up with the group, she was often in the lead right next to the guide, scrambling up challenging slopes. It was at dinner that night that her daughter Kim told us that Bette was 75 years old. I couldn't believe it. Bette looked and behaved far younger than that. As I spent more time chatting with her over the next couple of days, I became increasingly impressed with her positive attitude and easy-going manner.

At one point during a hike, as our group approached a summit, a couple of the other women and I were talking about how energetic Bette was. One woman said that her own mother had Alzheimer's. Another woman said that her mother always complained about aches and pains and never did anything physically active. I thought about my own mother who passed away in 1994 at a very young 60 years of age. I realized that if she were alive, she would have been the same age as Bette. We all walked in silence for a few minutes and I had to fight back the tears. I'm sure at that moment we each wished our mothers could be hiking with us, enjoying the sunshine and glorious scenery. I'm certain too that we all felt joy for Bette in that she could share the experience with her own daughter.

One day back at the lodge, Bette and Kim joined Allan and me in the hot tub. Then Kim, who happened to be a personal trainer and extremely fit, said she was going to jump into the pond next to the lodge to cool down. I couldn't believe that she did it. I then said I would do it too, and dared Allan to join me. Well, Bette chimed in that she would jump in the pond as well. I didn't think she would do it. Sure enough, Bette marched down to the pond with us and jumped right into the cold water. I was so impressed. It was a fun and memorable moment. Another time that Bette demonstrated her zest for life was at the end of our last hike when each of us had to zipline over a deep, rocky gorge. Bette had no fear. The guide hooked up her harness and off went Bette, zipping over the gorge.

I'll always remember Bette and what a remarkable inspiration she was. She unknowingly showed me and others what one can hope to become at an older age. After our trip was over and I was back home, I wrote Bette an email and told her what a true inspiration she was. I think it's important that when special people come into our lives, we let them know how they touched us. A few years later, I went to Arizona a couple of times to visit relatives. I made sure to contact Bette and get together. What did we do at our reunions? Why, we climbed mountains of course!

After the heli-hiking tour was over, Allan and I had a few days on our own in Banff, Alberta. I felt energized and wanted to do more physical activities, not just shopping and eating. We rented bicycles one day and cycled on paths in the mountains, enjoying a scenic picnic. There were some points along the paths when I couldn't get my bike up due to the steep inclines, so I got off my bike and pushed it up the hill. It was difficult but very enjoyable.

The final day of our trip, we did the unthinkable—white water rafting. Had someone told me a few months earlier that I would be hiking, ziplining, cycling in the mountains, and white water rafting, I would have said "No way!" But there we were, not on the gentle family float as I originally intended, but on class 4 rapids. In the raft I was flanked by a young U.S. marine who was soon being deployed to Iraq. I jokingly asked him to rescue me if I fell overboard. The whole ride was fun and thrilling. I was no longer a self-proclaimed chicken.

I was a warrior. I could do adventurous things. Hurray for me!

⤶⟶⟵⤷

Back from vacation, I wanted to continue doing active things. One evening when we were in the city, I took advantage of the flat terrain and decided to attempt a 12 kilometer run. I did it without difficulty. It took me 90 minutes. At that point, I realized that if I could run 12 kilometers, there was no reason I could not run a half marathon of 21.1 kilometers. It would just take longer. I had a steady pace, I didn't get out of breath, and my muscles didn't hurt. I'd either do the race in September or October, depending on how many practice opportunities I would have. The hilly runs I did at the cottage increased my physical stamina, but I needed longer runs to see if I had the mental stamina to go the distance.

As the end of August rolled around, I contemplated my successes and setbacks. Overall, I was proud that I had not regained weight during the summer. I had maintained a solid level of activity as evidenced by the entries in my daily exercise log that I'd started—a log which I continue to update all these years later. The days without any exercise were few and far between. I patted myself on the back for a job well done.

I'd progressed to 16-kilometer runs in under two hours—no small feat. My pace was faster, my strides were longer, and my lungs were stronger. In less than a month, I would be participating in my first half marathon.

Hard work pays off. It's an easy concept, but it's not always easy to execute. Consistency, perseverance, persistence, and a belief in yourself—that's what's required.

Suddenly, I just wasn't feeling it. I couldn't get myself to exercise regularly. It started when I was struck with a 12-hour bout of what I think was food poisoning. I had severe diarrhea overnight and was feeling weak the next day. I was being extra cautious about what I ate for a few days afterwards; therefore, I was not particularly energetic. So I took some time off from exercise and then it was hard to get back into it.

The latter part of August was outstanding in terms of the weather. Instead of taking advantage of that, I simply wanted to snooze on the dock and soak up the rays of sunshine that I craved. I

83

didn't feel like running or even stretching, which I had enjoyed doing all summer. I did a bit of this and that, but I just didn't have the energy to run the hills or do a full workout. Was I burned out?

After a week of slacking off, I was fed up with my behavior. I drove to the city to get in a long run. It started pouring rain as I arrived, so I had a decent hour-long workout at the gym instead. Then as the rain eased up and I couldn't stand the tedium of the treadmill, I headed outdoors for a run. I hadn't eaten a proper breakfast. A kilometer into my run, I was light-headed and needed to use the bathroom badly. I made a pit stop at Starbucks to use the facilities and then did some walk/run intervals to get back to the gym. Of course, it started raining again and I got soaked, but that didn't faze me. I felt disappointed with myself for being unable to run more than a couple of kilometers that day. Then I reminded myself that everyone is entitled to some downtime. The trick is to accept it and move forward.

⚘

By summer's end, I'd been writing this book for several months. I noticed that I had a bit of writer's block. The ideas were in me but I couldn't get the words into the computer as easily as before. I realized it was because what started out as a joke had turned into a meaningful journey. Exercise was no longer a laughing matter. Poking fun at myself and others was replaced by a seriousness that was driven by my now-established will to succeed. Insecurities and self-doubts that had plagued me months earlier were replaced by a new-found confidence. After all, I could climb mountains and raft through rapids with the toughest of the tough, and I was training for a half marathon.

I felt a sense of urgency to move forward with documenting my experiences and all that I'd learned. I toyed with the idea of someday sharing my story with those who need guidance and inspiration. And so, my writing took on a more serious note that reflected my feelings. I deleted the original, tongue-in-cheek title for my book—*Shut Your Mouth and Move Your Ass: This Bitch Has the Real Skinny On How to Get Fit*—and I replaced it with the current title.

⚘

On August 29, 2008, I hit another milestone. I checked my weight at the gym and was shocked that I was down to 135 pounds. This was just about what I weighed nine years earlier when I got pregnant with my second son—only now I was leaner and stronger. Frankly, I never thought I'd be able to get to that weight again since I was now approaching my 45th birthday. It goes to show you that with reasonable eating habits and regular exercise, you can regain your former body—even an improved version of it!

Labor Day came and went. We moved back to the city. The kids went back to school and I got back into my daily gym routine. I did the cardio kickboxing class that I'd missed. The instructor had us doing flying kicks, with both feet in the air at the same time. It was fun. It was tough. It was a much harder workout than I'd done all summer. I also worked out on my own with weights that morning. In the evening, I decided I had to try another long run because the day of the half marathon was fast approaching. I put on a new pair of lightweight running shorts that I'd just purchased, my compression sports bra, a tank top, my dual-layer running socks, and my running shoes which were still giving me blisters when I ran. By now those blisters were turning into callouses, giving me "runner's feet," as my friend Anna the marathon queen informed me. A cool, gentle breeze and a slowly setting sun were the perfect accompaniments for my run. I never felt better running. I ran 19 kilometers and was delighted as I arrived home at 9:30 p.m. engulfed in darkness and drenched in sweat. I had regained my confidence and knew I could do the half marathon in just over two weeks, come hell or high water.

In the past, when I had an opportunity to try something new, I'd often give it minimal consideration before dismissing it. Now I was jumping at such opportunities, so when Gina asked me to join her for some Yin yoga, I decided to give it a try. I had only been to a yoga class once before and had found it to be extremely boring. Gina took me to a yoga studio where we lay on mats awaiting the instructor. We joked around in hushed voices and I wondered how on earth I was going to stop giggling when the class started. The instructor arrived and announced that this was a 90-minute class. Yikes! Ninety minutes of holding torturous poses? What if I couldn't do it? It turned out that I was fully capable. We held each pose for several minutes with our eyes closed, focusing on our breathing. I found Yin yoga very relaxing. It was great to try something new.

❧

    I had plans to attend a fundraising event and I had one pair of dressy slacks that I thought would fit me. I had tried them on a few weeks prior. I tried them on the day before the event and they were so loose on my rear end and hips that I looked like a pickle floating in a barrel. I didn't have anything appropriate to wear so I headed to the mall, credit card in hand. I went to a nice shop and tried on size 10 tweed slacks. They were huge! So I tried on size 8. Still way too big. The sales clerk handed me a size 6 and they almost fit, just a bit too snug. So I went to another store and tried on some nice skirts, also size 6. Everything fit beautifully. As I inspected myself in the full-length mirror on the outside of the fitting room door, the sales women fawned over me. I thought to myself, "Wow! I look great." My stomach looked so flat, my boobs looked high and perky (thanks to the new bra I was wearing), and I felt very happy. I felt like I was on a hidden camera show and people were replacing the size tags on the clothing to trick me into thinking I was size 6. I couldn't believe it. It felt good! On another day, I went shopping for jeans. I tried on jeans in a size 30-inch waist. They were huge. I tried on 29 and still loose. A 28-inch waist, could it be true? Yes! Again I was surprised at the new size I needed and how much fun shopping was when everything looked good on me. No more tummy bulge to contend with. No more having to suck in my gut in order to zip the pants. I was loving every minute of it and wondered how much my physical transformation was going to cost in terms of assembling a new wardrobe.

    I continued to receive compliments wherever I went. Enough with the compliments already. But they kept coming, from other moms at school pickup; from the make-up artist at the mall who told me I looked very athletic and asked me for some weight-loss tips; from the young man who worked at my children's music school and who asked me what I was eating and what exercises I was doing; from the Asian aesthetician who, while massaging my calves during a pedicure remarked, "You have big muksles," referring in her broken English to my calf muscles; and from the saleswoman at a boutique who, when I stood in front of the mirror to see how I looked in a short dress, declared, "You must work out a lot. Look at your legs!" It never stopped. Several times a day I would get compliments and questions about how I did it.

One day, I posted a photo of myself on my Facebook profile. It was a photo of me in a bodybuilder type of pose, jokingly flexing my biceps while wearing a bikini. Within a day, I had friends writing that I looked buff and hot. One commented, "You are looking fabulous—I'm truly in awe of your dedication to healthy living and the results are very obvious!" Another friend wrote, "This photo will get you many hot dates. Your husband should be proud to have such a fox like you!" After a couple of days, I decided to remove the photo, but the compliments and attention had been fun.

Before I knew it, there was just one week to go until my first half marathon. I was going to ease off on the running and other forms of exercise that last week so as not to injure myself or have sore muscles on race day. I would do a couple of short runs, which for me now meant an 8 and a 5 kilometer run. Funny, just three months prior, I had found 5 kilometers to be very challenging. Now anything fewer than 10 kilometers seemed like a short run. My body and mind had become acclimated to the demands of running. I just hoped that on race day my body and mind would make it to the finish line. Persist and persevere. I'm not sure if I coined that phrase or if I heard or read it somewhere, but it became one of my running mantras. When I had to push through a wall such as muscle fatigue or energy depletion, I would say to myself repeatedly, "Persist and persevere." That would get me past the wall.

Some of my friends were asking me if I was getting excited about race day. My response, for some reason, was "not really." I think I didn't want to get excited because I was a bit concerned that I may not finish the run and I would disappoint friends who had encouraged me in recent months; more importantly, I would disappoint myself. That was probably just nerves as the race day fast approached. I worried that I might have bathroom issues during the half marathon. An urgent need to use the facilities had plagued me on recent long runs. In the summer, the woods were my companion, offering me a constantly available and much appreciated area of privacy. In the city it was a different matter. On my last long run a week and a half before race day, I had a moment of desperation. I feared I would have no recourse but to take a dump in the bushes behind a church. Even though I'm Jewish, that option was undeniably sacrilegious. Fortunately, I was able to hold on until I got to Starbucks. Ah, Starbucks—the best latté after a good workout and the most cherished bathroom during a run.

I knew there would be porta potties on the half marathon course, but I was praying that I'd be able to complete the race without cramps or a sudden uncontrollable urge to go when there would be no porta potty in sight. I felt confident that the distance per se would not be a problem. My body had gotten used to the force of my feet hitting the pavement for two and a half hours. During training runs, I experienced a few muscle aches in my quads and calves, but nothing I couldn't run through. All I wished for was an empty bowel and decent weather; the rest I could manage.

Four days before the half marathon, I did my last training run of 7 kilometers as I powered down. It felt great doing a short run. There was a cool breeze and it was sunny. I was feeling confident again and looking forward to the big day and to the emotional high of crossing the finish line.

I read a book entitled *What I Talk About When I Talk About Running* (2009), an inspirational memoir written by a man who took up marathon running as a lifelong hobby. The author described his challenges, lessons learned, and the thrill of achievement. I soaked up his words of wisdom and realized that I now considered myself "a runner." I don't just run. I am a runner!

⚮

Thirty-six hours before my anticipated finish, I lay in bed and looked at the clock. It was midnight. I was anxious. I felt the adrenaline coursing through my veins. Earlier that day, a friend had dropped off a newspaper article that she'd written 15 years earlier. In it, she described her experience running the Boston Marathon, and how she openly wept as she approached the finish line. Attached to the article was a thoughtful, handwritten note wishing me good luck on my run.

As I lay in bed, I thought about her triumph and imagined my own moment of glory, which was just hours away. All the steps of my physical and emotional journey of the past year up until this time, and all the people who helped me and believed in me whizzed through my mind. Every milestone, big and small, and every person who made a difference, big or small, appeared one after another like a fast-forwarded slideshow in my mind.

I started to quietly weep as I realized that in a few hours I would be rushing towards the finish line. That would be the culmination of a year's worth of effort. It was exactly one year to the day, September 21, 2007, that Gina had taken my measurements and jotted them down, at my request, on a piece of paper that I'd since kept tucked away in my jewellery box. The numbers on that piece of paper helped me remember how far I'd travelled on my journey. It was exactly one year from the day I finally decided to do something and get fit, to the day of the half marathon. Seven inches off my waist, over 20 pounds off my body, and I was feeling fit and fantastic. I was ready for the run of my life!

Unable to sleep, I tossed and turned. I thought about several special people who believed in me even when I wasn't quite ready to believe in myself. I imagined the words of gratitude I wished to offer each of them. I vividly recalled details of conversations and email exchanges in which these people encouraged me to pursue my half marathon goal. The first person who came to mind was Lynne. She'd been one of the first people to whom I declared my goal of running a half marathon. I remembered how her email reply included, "I have no doubt you'll achieve your goal." She never expressed doubt or questioned my ability. Those few words of confidence from someone I truly admired helped me believe I could really do it. From that moment onwards, I knew that if I trained hard and well, I could complete the race.

I also recalled the time my friend Anna, the experienced marathoner, told me she was going to wait at the 20 kilometer point so she could cheer me on as I got to that last and potentially toughest kilometer of the run. I was really touched that she would be there for me. She assured me that I would indeed complete the run and even suggested that maybe next year I should aim for a full marathon. She never doubted me. It felt great to have believers.

All the people at my gym who heard about my upcoming race and who wished me well came to mind. Tears continued to stream down my cheeks. Maybe it was the anticipation coupled with intense gratitude and some nerves. So many emotions. Finally, sleep engulfed me.

⁊⁊⁊

The day before the race, I went with Allan and the boys to pick up my race kit. It included a souvenir technical running shirt and a timing chip for my shoe. The race was called The Canada Army Run. It was the inaugural race. There were military personnel and veterans as well as several military vehicles on display. The run would include both a half marathon and a 5 kilometer race. Participants registered for the 5 kilometer race got white shirts. Those of us registered for the half marathon got black shirts. I pulled my black shirt over my T-shirt and proudly walked about, feeling athletic and proud. Now I was more excited. I wanted to run right then and there. I could hardly wait. I felt a great sense of pride being a half marathoner.

Sunday, September 20, 2008—Race day came and went in the blink of an eye. I remember the sense of excitement as I stepped over the start line and got into a comfortable pace. It was a cool, overcast day, just perfect for me. No hot sun beating down on me. I felt good. No bathroom emergencies either! The race started at 9 a.m. but I'd been up since 5 a.m. to ensure I had a good breakfast and was hydrated. I gave myself plenty of time to sit and relax in the washroom. I expected to finish the run anywhere from 2 hours and 30 minutes as a best-case scenario, to 2 hours and 45 minutes.

I was amazed at the variety of ages, sizes, and shapes of the runners. Lots of ordinary people doing extraordinary things. I'll never forget the disabled army veteran with the long scar on his skull riding his specially outfitted bike. I chatted just before the race with a woman named Becky from Pembroke, Ontario. I later saw her half-way through and we waved to each other. There are many people who I will never know by name that I must thank. Thanks to all the folks who cheered for the runners. Thanks to the little boy with the "high five" sign whom many of us high-fived. Thanks to the loud-mouthed runner whose voice and ridiculous banter with his group of runners was so annoying that I found myself increasing my pace just to get away from him. Thanks to the young lady ahead of me in line for the porta potty who promised to get in and out in record time and delivered on her promise. Thanks to Allan, Jesse, and Joshua for surprising me at the 15 kilometer mark with a "Go Glo" sign and loving smiles that nearly brought me to tears, and for waiting for me at the finish line.

It was tough, my legs were sore, and it was exhausting, but I felt elated during the whole run. I sprinted towards the finish line with a big smile on my face. It was definitely not as difficult as I had thought it would be. I surprised myself. I felt great afterwards as well and was delighted to share my victory with my family. I'll cherish for a long time to come the army tag medallion that I was handed as I crossed the finish line. It may only be worth a few cents, but to me it represents a year's worth of effort and determination. I learned something about myself that day: There are many things in life I'd never do for any price; but dangle a piece of tin on a toilet chain and I'll run 21.1 kilometers for it!

I completed my first half marathon in 2 hours 33 minutes and 7 seconds. I was so happy with my result. Except for a few minutes at the porta potty, I ran the whole thing straight through, slow and steady. And even though I was in the bottom 10 percent of all runners and the bottom 15 percent of women in my age group of 40 to 49, it didn't matter to me. I achieved my goal, I exceeded my personal expectations, and I felt terrific. Next time—and as soon as the race was over I was already certain there would be a next time—I would try to improve on my "PB." I learned that PB means Personal Best. Oooh, I love talking running jargon.

❧❧❧

When I think back to that day, and especially to that moment when I crossed the finish line, I realize that it's not the destination, but the journey, that is most special. It sounds cliché, but it's true. I cherish each little moment of glory: the first time I ran more than 5 kilometers without stopping; the time I ran to the mailbox and back and pushed myself with every ounce of effort to get up those killer hills as my heart raced and my thighs burned; all those city runs to Starbucks and back and beyond as I increased my distance and tested my mental and physical endurance; the mini milestones, the aches and bathroom emergencies, having to repeat my mantra to get through difficult moments, and having to remind myself or convince myself that I am a warrior.

I'd walked the path of diamonds that Robin Sharma described in *The Monk Who Sold His Ferrari*. I'd embraced life. I felt happy and fulfilled. Sometimes getting to the destination is an anticlimax. Crossing that finish line meant that all my training had paid off, that all my sweat equity had been a worthwhile investment.

As extreme runner Ray Zahab, whose many incredible exploits include running across the Sahara Desert, explained in his book *Running for My Life*, "My limits were all in my mind…Once you go beyond what you ever thought you could do, there's no going back. It's with you forever" (p. 138).

Zahab's sentiments resonated with me. I'd pushed the boundaries of my abilities. Crossing the finish line was a defining moment in my life. I realized that this accomplishment was now a part of who I'd become. No one would ever be able to take that away! Looking back at all of my achievements, the half marathon was probably the most difficult thing I'd ever done. In my mind, I was like my inspiration, Ray Zahab, who also changed his lifestyle and took up running later in life. In different ways, we'd each improved our lives and become different people.

The day after the half marathon, I was feeling great. No aches or pains. I was back into my normal workout routine at the gym. I wore my dog tag medal but kept it tucked under my shirt, showing it only to those who asked to see it. Everyone was surprised at how well I felt. I received so much positive feedback from my peers. I wondered what my next goal would be. I decided to wait a while before writing some new goals. I wanted to bask in the glory of my accomplishment. Three days after the run, I felt the urge to run again. It felt good to be out there with my feet hitting the pavement, on my own with my thoughts.

Personal Best Exercises

o   What risks are you willing to take to improve your fitness and health?

o   Think of a physical activity or an active adventure you'd like to pursue, and then create a plan for how you can make it happen.

o   Practice thinking positive, empowering thoughts every day. Begin by writing a positive affirmation on a piece of paper and stick it on your bathroom mirror so you can read it every time you brush your teeth.

Did you know?

• A daily weigh-in can keep you on track. On the other hand, daily weigh-ins can become obsessive, and daily fluctuations can be discouraging. Some people prefer to weigh themselves once a week. Whatever you choose to do, remember that body composition is more important than body weight.

• Investing a bit of time at the start of each week will help you remain in maintenance mode. Plan and prepare meals and snacks for home and on the go. Plan your weekly exercise schedule and make it non-negotiable. Remember to make your health and wellness a top priority so you don't fall back into a pattern that deters you from your goals.

• One of the secrets for long-term maintenance is to find your passion. Find a sport or type of exercise that makes your face light up when you think or talk about it. Find something you love and look forward to doing. When you find something that excites you, you'll feel motivated to work hard at it and develop that passion. Invest time, energy, and resources into your passion. In what currency will you measure the return on your investment? You'll measure it in health and happiness.

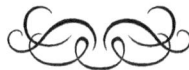

PART II

SONGS OF TRANSFORMATION

8 REVOLUTION

I made up my mind there and then that I was not going to give up.

A week after the half marathon, I felt ready to try something new. I'd recently been looking at roller blades at the mall. They were on sale but I was reluctant to buy a pair since I had only tried roller blading once. Actually, it was roller skating at the roller disco back then, over 30 years ago. The new style roller blades, also known as inline skates, look very different from the roller skates of my childhood and they require different skating techniques. I felt a bit intimidated. What if I fall? What if I injure myself? Worse, what if I looked like a klutz?

I reminded myself that I was supposed to have no fear. I borrowed my nephew's roller blades and decided to give it a whirl. Lynne offered to show me how to roller blade. That was an offer I couldn't refuse. She was an avid roller blader and I knew she wouldn't laugh at me.

I sat on her front steps and strapped on the roller blades. I put on my son's skateboard helmet and velcroed on some wrist and knee guards. All I remember after that is Lynne roller blading down her slanted driveway beckoning me to join her. I was still sitting on her steps shouting, "Wait for me!" I didn't know how to stand up on those suckers, how to get moving, or how to balance. Worst of all, I didn't know what I didn't know—and that was how to stop. Lynne went ahead and shouted for me to follow her. And so I did just that. I got up, got my balance, pushed off, and voila—I was roller blading. Woo hoo! Within a few minutes, I was rolling along fairly comfortably. I unclenched my fists and began to relax. This wasn't so bad!

Suddenly, a car came down the road right towards me. How do I stop?! The rear brake was counterintuitive and I just couldn't get the hang of it, so I slowed down by rolling off to the side of the road at an angle, then I stepped onto a lawn. Phew! Not that bad. It would be better if I could brake, but hey, you can't master every skill all on the first attempt.

It's never too late to learn a new sport or skill. A couple of days later, I went by myself to the park in my neighbourhood. I roller bladed along the walking paths. There were no cars to potentially kill me, and few pedestrians for me to potentially knock over. I roller bladed around the paths for nearly an hour, enjoying the cool autumn breeze and the warm sun. As the wheels revolved, I felt like I was undergoing a revolution.

One day, I drove a few miles away to the Ottawa River. People go there to cycle, walk, run, and roller blade on the paths. The pavement there is smooth and crack-free and the views are rather scenic. I listened to music on my iPod. I felt comfortable and was going much faster than usual, with longer glides.

I had another epiphany. I felt as though, in a sense, I'd wasted many precious years trapped indoors when I worked full time. I had worked in one of the coveted corner offices with large windows from which I used to peer out on sunny days and wish I were somewhere else—like a bird in a gilded cage. As I roller bladed smoothly along the path and enjoyed the scenery, the fresh air and the warmth of the sun on my face, I thought that everyone should spend more time doing the things they enjoy. I felt blessed to have so much freedom.

<hr>

As my self-confidence and physical strength continued to increase, I decided to try an abdominal exercise that I'd seen in a women's fitness magazine. It was a hanging leg lift in which you hold onto an overhead bar and raise your legs upwards as high as you can until you're in a pike position. I'd actually tried this exercise a few months earlier, but I'd only been able to lift my legs 90 degrees. This time, I was able to bring my legs completely straight up and lower and raise them in this manner a few times per set. According to the magazine article, in order to make this exercise an extreme challenge that few women (and probably few men) could do, I needed to not only go into a pike position, but then to rotate my legs from side to side while keeping them together. This was called the windshield wiper. That would be my next goal— to work on mastering the windshield wiper move. I needed to strengthen my abdominal muscles, in particular my obliques, to be able to do that.

As I practiced the exercise at the gym, people would look at me in amazement. After a while, I no longer found it very difficult. I was getting stronger abs. Some of my friends saw me and attempted the exercise. They tried to raise their legs and could barely raise them 45 degrees. I felt strong and fit and I wondered how long it would be until I could do the side-to-side windshield wiper motion.

A woman approached me at the gym one day. She told me she was impressed with the variety of challenging exercises she'd seen me do. She also seemed very fit. I'd noticed her doing some tough exercises as well. Over time, we ended up engaged in a friendly competition to see who could do more leg raises, chin-ups, and push-ups. Sometimes we sent each other encouraging notes on Facebook and she thanked me for showing her how to do some exercises. I felt terrific knowing that in some small way I inspired her. She inspired me too.

One day, I noticed a bright red boxing bag set up in the gym. It was exactly like mine—the one I'd been using at the cottage. The boxing bag at the gym was usually kept under lock and key and I had never seen anyone use it before. The room in which fitness classes were conducted was being renovated, so all of the equipment from its closets was out in the main exercise room. I happened to have my boxing gloves in my backpack, as I sometimes wore them during cardio kickboxing classes even though that was a non-contact class. I knew I should put on my protective hand wraps under my gloves, as I always did when I boxed at my cottage, but I didn't have them with me and I figured I'd just practice a few light punches on the bag.

As soon as I started warming up with some light jabs, it seemed that all eyes were on me. A senior gentleman, who was a regular at the gym, egged me on to punch and kick harder. I told him I was just warming up and we both laughed. He continued to watch me. Once I warmed up, I started practicing a variety of combinations that included the jab, cross, hook, and upper cut as well as front and side kicks. As I got into it, I packed more power into my punches.

After a few minutes, I took off my gloves to air out my hands and I noticed some redness between my fingers. I dismissed it as dye from the gloves since my hands were so sweaty. I got a drink of water then put my gloves back on and continued kickboxing. I was really working up a sweat. I felt a bit self-conscious since I was not only making noises as my gloves made contact with the bag, but I was also grunting as I turned my body into the bag and drove my crosses and hooks with increasing force. The cardio kickboxing instructor had always encouraged his students to breathe properly and make some noise to get more power. I was concerned that I might be disturbing people who were working out, but I was having a great workout and really enjoying myself. I didn't want to stop.

In a way, I felt like I was putting on a show. This was probably the first time anyone had ever boxed in that room and possibly the first time some of the people there had seen a woman hit a bag.

When I was done, I took off my gloves and did some abdominal exercises and stretches before heading home. My knuckles felt a little bit sore. When I arrived home, I noticed they were terribly bruised, tender, and swollen, especially on my right hand, which is my dominant hand. I looked as though I had been in a brawl. It was a day before the swelling went down and the black and blue began to fade. I'm lucky I didn't have more serious damage. I learned a couple of valuable lessons: always gear up properly and never underestimate your own power.

Later that day, I finished reading *What I Talk About When I Talk About Running*. In describing his experiences with marathons and triathlons, author Haruki Murakami says, "It's precisely because of the pain, precisely because we want to overcome that pain, that we can get the feeling, through this process, of really being *alive*—or at least a partial sense of it. Your quality of experience is based not on standards such as time and ranking, but on finally awakening to an awareness of the fluidity within action itself" (p. 171).

I understood what Murakami meant. Whatever sport or exercise I engaged in, for me it was not about competing against others; rather, I was constantly trying to improve myself and I felt awakened and aware of what I was doing. Whether I was running, hitting a boxing bag, or drawing on all my strength to get my legs up into a pike position, I was energized by the action itself. If an occasional minor pain was the side-effect, then so be it. I could overcome the pain if that was the price of feeling a sense of aliveness.

❧

Over the course of about a week, I purged my basement of approximately 14 years' worth of accumulated junk, from small kitchen appliances that no longer worked properly, to numerous toys and odds and sods. It was very cleansing to get rid of all that junk. I then emptied the guest bedroom, which we rarely needed. I converted that room into my personal home gym. I put my exercise ball, dumbbells, mini trampoline, and mat in it. I had brought my boxing bag back from the cottage and moved it into my gym. I hung up my running medals and race bibs on a bulletin board. I plugged in my CD player so I could listen to energizing music during workouts and relaxing music during stretching. I bought incense so I could have some scent (other than body odor) for meditation. Even though that room was windowless, I felt happy in it. It was clean, uncluttered, and all mine. I put my name plate, which I had kept after I was laid off from my job, on the door. I boxed to my heart's content that evening, then stretched on the mat. Fragrant incense permeated the room. My sweet escape.

❧

One day in late October, I awoke to another beautiful cool, crisp autumn morning. I had been thinking about participating in a 10 kilometer race organized by Mothers Against Drunk Drivers (MADD). Since the weather was perfect, I jumped out of bed, got ready, and headed out to the run site for the MADD Dash. This was a timed event and all finishers were to receive a medal, which was a big incentive for me.

I enjoyed a pleasant run through a suburban neighbourhood. The fall colors were so pretty. I felt a bit weary around the 8-kilometer mark, but I pushed myself to run a bit faster. I sprinted the last few hundred meters. I finished in 1:04:18. I was happy with that time. Allan and the kids surprised me by meeting me at the finish line.

Runners love statistics. My identity as a runner strengthened with each race and I, too, became increasingly eager to check my stats online as soon as I got home. For this race, my pace was my personal best. I placed 44th out of 73 women and 87th out of all 119 participants.

I started googling to find half marathons in the southern United States that I was hoping would coincide with one of the winter school breaks. Maybe I could fit a race into an upcoming family vacation? I recognized that thought as a sign that I was becoming obsessed with running.

⚘

Three days after I participated in the MADD Dash, an old high school classmate—with whom I'd reconnected via Facebook after losing touch in 1981—posted a shocking announcement on her Facebook page. Her sister had been killed by a drunk driver. How awful. Her sister had been confined to a wheelchair after suffering from polio as a child. While out and about in her Montreal neighbourhood on her 47th birthday, she was struck by a repeat offender and found lifeless in a ditch. What a tragedy. Life can end at any time, so it seems. All the more reason to try to live each day to the fullest.

⚘

Back at the gym, the manager approached me to ask if I'd be interested in taking courses to get certified as a fitness instructor or, specifically, as a kickboxing instructor. I was flattered, but I wasn't interested in starting a new career. I enjoyed not working. But the idea of sharing my passion for fitness with other people was appealing. Perhaps I'd pursue certification in the new year. For now, I'd think about it.

⚘

I continued to receive compliments from people at least once a day. It was so odd. "What's your secret?" asked a senior at my gym. He had known me 20 years ago when I was friends with his daughter. He told me I looked great and wanted to know how I did it. I told him my secret was to stop eating at fast-food restaurants several times per week like I used to do. One of the mothers with whom I chatted at school pickup told me I was getting "skinny." I asked her how she could tell since I was wearing a large winter coat. She said she saw me running the week before.

"I'm not trying to get skinny, just fit," I remarked with a wink.

⤫

I had another formal fundraising event coming up. I splurged on a gorgeous new outfit, only to be informed by my former personal trainer Gina, who'd become my friend, that it was too formal for the occasion. I thought the long, black ruffled skirt and the black and white embroidered jacket were classy and sophisticated. I felt elegant modeling the outfit for Gina until she burst my bubble and said it was suitable for a 60-year-old woman, not for me. She suggested we go shopping together. I'm not sure why I listened to her. First we stopped at her house where she showed me the dress she was going to wear to the gala. I thought to myself, "Is that a slip? Where's the rest of the outfit?" It was a sheer, very short dress with spaghetti straps. I asked her what type of bra would go with that dress and she told me she was going to go braless in it. I couldn't believe it. I told her I could never wear something like that. And braless? Was she serious?! She was pushing 50. The last time I went braless, I was 12. It just didn't seem appropriate, at least not by my standards. Gina laughed and said I have a great figure and should show it off.

I realized it takes time to get used to one's new figure after losing weight and shaping up. I went shopping with Gina. Despite her attempt to convince me to show more skin, I ended up buying a knee-length, black, sleeveless dress with a high neckline. I didn't impress Gina with my rather conservative selection, but I felt it was right for me.

As one of our mutual friends later told me, after I described Gina's skimpy dress, "Never shop for clothes with someone who has the body of a Playboy centerfold."

Maybe I was being too self-conscious or lacking in self-esteem despite my significant physical improvements over the past year. Even when I was much younger and very slim, I never was the type to wear revealing clothing. We each have our own comfort level. And so I'd wear my somewhat modest but attractive dress to the event. I'd accessorize it with diamonds, a martini, and my handsome husband on my arm.

By the time the next formal event came up several months later, I'd gained the confidence to wear something that revealed a bit more of my new and hard-earned body. I wore a short, low-cut, figure-hugging red dress that made me stand out from the black-tie crowd. I definitely felt like a sexy mama. Allan and I were among the many couples who took turns posing for a photo in front of a black grand piano. The photographer asked each couple how they'd like to pose. Unlike everyone else, I spontaneously jumped up on the piano and lay across it, with Allan standing next to the piano looking sharp in his tuxedo.

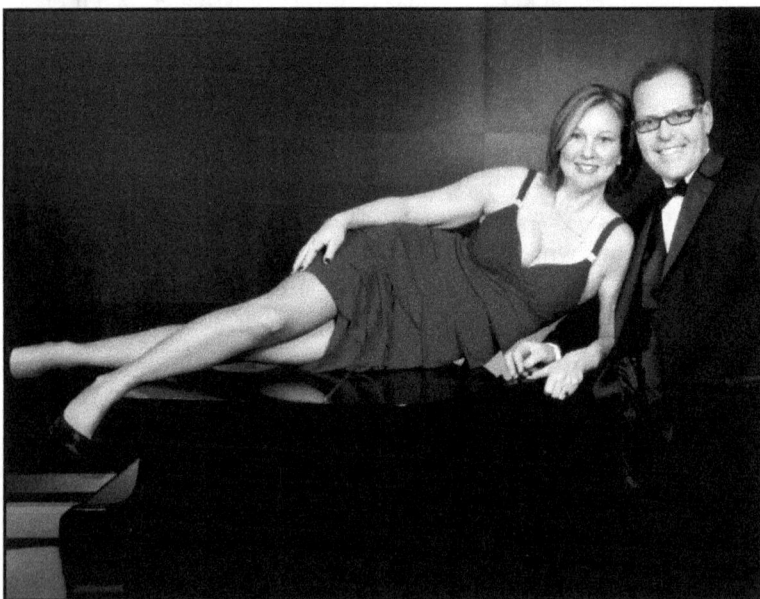

Posing on a grand piano next to Allan. I felt proud to display my new physique and my new attitude. (Photo by Valberg Imaging)

A day of downtime is a good thing. It allows the body time to recover from a hard workout. A day of being lazy and eating garbage is a totally different ball game. I awoke one morning feeling like I really had to move. I'd overslept. I'd eaten a chocolate bar, cheesies, and ice cream the day before. I hadn't exercised. I felt gross. Now I was itching to be active.

It was a crisp but sunny late November morning. I put on several layers of clothes including wicking long johns and a matching undershirt, winter running pants, a jersey, and a fleece vest. I also donned my new winter running hat and some gloves. I headed out for my standard 8 kilometer run. Man, it was cold! I think it was minus seven Celsius, but with the wind chill it felt much colder. My sunglasses fogged up immediately and my lungs took in cold air. I tucked my glasses into my pocket and kept going.

"I am a warrior," I reminded myself. Within a few minutes, I was warmed up except for my nose, cheeks and gloved fingers, which felt the sting of the biting cold. I felt proud to be out in this challenging weather. I felt tough pushing my limits. Because I had a bathroom emergency on the way, I made a pit stop at Starbucks and then decided to stay for a hot drink. I used to order coffee drinks containing sweetened syrup and whipped cream—lots of unnecessary calories. I gave those up and switched to a better choice—a decaf, non-fat latté. I warmed up and read the Sunday newspaper for 45 minutes. I never stop for coffee on a run but it was so darn cold out. I needed to warm myself from the inside out. Eventually, I got up out of my comfy chair. As I was heading out the door, preparing to walk home the four kilometers, a young woman looked at me with admiration.

"I wish I could get out in this weather and run," she remarked. Well, that was just what I needed to hear. No walking home for this warrior. I ran home and felt rejuvenated.

Later that day, I took Joshua to see the animated Disney movie *Bolt*. It features a hamster character that dreams about being a superhero. When the other characters mock him, he maintains his upbeat attitude and retorts, "The impossible is possible when you're awesome!" I love that line. I wanted to have an attitude like that hamster. Maybe I already did.

Gloria Schwartz

November had been a difficult month in terms of sticking to healthy eating. I'd attended two bar mitzvahs, each of which included an extravagant catered buffet lunch and dinner with sweet tables. I'd also attended a couple of fundraising galas with delicious food and decadent desserts, appetizers, and cocktails. There were also some extra restaurant dinners for friends' birthdays. At each event, I tried to think before I ate, but I did want to enjoy myself. I was pretty good considering the smorgasbord of delectable treats that confronted me. I was able to maintain some sense of self-control and resist much of the sweet table offerings. I resisted the fried appetizers. For the sit-down dinners, I ate half of what was on my plate and had a few bites of desserts. Still, all the extra calories and fat (not to mention the sodium) was more than I would have normally consumed and probably more than I was burning off.

If all that wasn't bad enough, I'd also recently indulged in chocolate-covered almonds. I'd purchased a party-size package to serve when some friends came over. After the get-together, I kept dipping into them. I had very little willpower when snacks were in the house. Even though I would take a respectable handful of the chocolate almonds, I'd go back for seconds and thirds. That was the problem. The original portion size was fine. One has to live a little and enjoy, right? However, the lack of self-control and that imaginary little voice in the cupboard calling my name were the vestiges of the old Gloria that I still couldn't completely shake. Once an addict, always an addict? As I ate another handful of chocolate almonds, I'd tell myself that I'd had enough, they were too sweet, they weren't good for my health, and that I wasn't really enjoying them, yet I kept munching on them.

Two weeks down the road, I'd be heading off for a family vacation in the Mayan Riviera in Mexico. An all-inclusive week of fun in the sun with unlimited food and drinks. I wasn't worried about the alcohol since I hardly drank. I would have to mentally prepare myself or else I would end up eating ice cream at lunch and cake at supper. I knew this because I'd done this in the past at resorts. When the food is there and it's all included, it's more tempting than ever. I'd make a plan to hit the gym and do some outdoor running and yoga on the beach every day to fill my time. If I only lay by the pool or on the beach, I'd have more time per day to stuff my face. If I worked out daily, I'd feel more inclined to watch what I eat. That was my plan.

Hopefully, it would work. One of my friends jokingly advised me to lay on my back by the pool the whole time I'd be on vacation; in doing so, she said my stomach would appear flat even if I over-indulged. Good plan, except what happens when I stand up?

⁂

I had a temporary moment of insanity one evening after speaking with an acquaintance about running. I went online and signed up for a half marathon, which is not that big a deal considering I'd done one already. The big deal was that this one takes place in Ottawa in late February, the coldest time of the year. I thought it would motivate me to keep up my running through winter. After registering for the half marathon, I enthusiastically laid out my winter running gear and was planning an 8 kilometer run for the next day. My enthusiasm was extinguished as soon as I stuck my nose out the door in the morning. It was snowing heavily and it was a cold -13 degrees Celsius. My goal of completing a half marathon in late February would hopefully get me going again early in the new year. I intended on training even if it meant freezing my butt off. If I could do a second half marathon, especially under intense conditions, then I could start training after that for a full marathon in May.

⁂

On December 1, I proved to myself that the impossible is possible. I was at the gym and the weight benches were occupied, so I decided to do a couple of chin-ups first. I had always done chin-ups after my upper-body workout. On this day, I was able to do two sets of four chin-ups.

Chin-ups are difficult, especially for women, because we have less upper body strength. Interestingly, more than half of the female recruits in the United States Marine Corps' boot camp failed the 2014 new fitness requirement to perform three chin-ups, and these are women half my age! I felt miraculously strong and it felt like my body was almost weightless. I felt like I had super powers like the animated hamster. From that point on, I'd do my chin-ups at the start of my workouts. By building strength and applying a better strategy, I had surpassed my goal.

≈

December went by quickly. Our trip to the hot and sunny Mayan Riviera gave me a well-needed energy boost. I followed through with my plan to exercise on my trip. I jogged early in the morning before it got too hot, I worked out at the resort's fitness center, and I ran laps in the pool for an hour each day. For the first time in many years, I felt comfortable walking around in a bikini. I felt very fit.

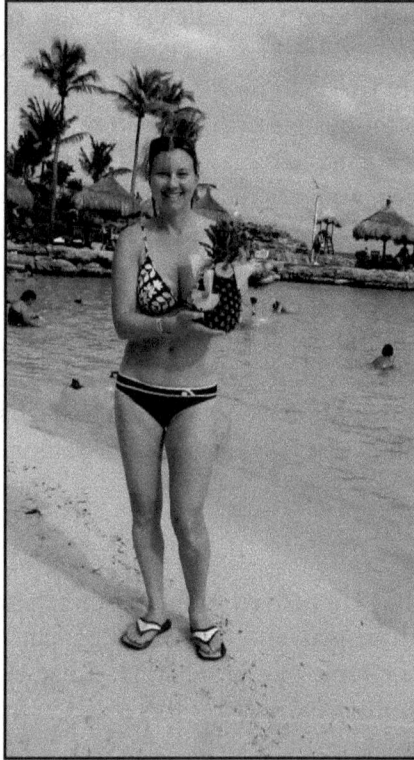

All the hard work had paid off. I was about to turn 45, yet my abs were flatter than they'd been in 20 years and stronger than ever.

The problem, as I'd expected, was with the food. After the first day, I succumbed to the temptations. The variety and quantity of available food was enticing. I had a few cocktails here and there and ate larger portions than I eat at home. I also indulged in desserts—my Achilles' heel.

After the trip, I worked out almost every day during the rest of the holiday break. I also returned to normal portions and less fattening foods. It had been fun to indulge, but I felt better eating properly. The two pounds I'd gained on vacation melted off. I celebrated my 45th birthday on December 31, 2008. I felt terrific.

✧

Allan and I took Jesse and Joshua on a four-day trip to Manhattan in late January. We had been sightseeing and shopping when we arrived at the edge of Central Park at 5th Avenue and 58th Street. It was a cool day but much warmer than Ottawa, so I felt energized and excited about the prospect of running in the Big Apple. I handed Allan my heavy leather jacket. He took the boys to look at the ice skaters and I took off for a short run. I had my music playing on my iPod. I looked up at the skyscrapers surrounding the park. I took in a deep breath of New York City air. James Blunt's melodic song *1973* started to play. I felt lucky to be alive and to be enjoying the view and the overall experience.

I was amazed at myself, quite frankly, because since I'd become a self-proclaimed fitness warrior, vacations now included physical fitness. Years ago, I'd travelled many times to New York. Back then, it never crossed my mind to run. Now running was a part of me and I wanted to experience it wherever I went. It was exciting running in different cities—the views, the people, the smells, the sounds. Each location provided me with a different experience that fulfilled my inexplicable need to run somewhere new. Perhaps that desire is part of the runner's psyche.

✧

By late February, I'd only run outdoors sporadically. Now I had to face the music—the Winterman Race was just around the corner and I was registered for the half marathon. I really wanted to do it but knew realistically I could not, or at least, I could not without risk of injury due to my lack of winter training. I decided I still wanted to participate, so I switched from the half marathon to the 10 km race. I knew I could pull off a 10K in the winter.

The morning after a fun-filled dinner party with Allan, my trainer friends and their partners, I woke up feeling parched. Gina's husband had poured a very strong gin and tonic that I'd enjoyed, but that I was unaccustomed to. I'd only slept about three hours. I dreamed I ran the race and was not awarded a finisher's medal because I'd forgotten to wear a timing chip. After that dream, I was anxious and tossed and turned for two hours. I got out of bed around 6 a.m. I was psyched for the race. I rehydrated myself and ate a light breakfast. Allan drove me to the Canadian War Museum and dropped me off. The roads looked dry so I made a last-minute decision to check my anti-slip shoe crampons into the baggage check area. Fatal error. Several minutes into the run, it started to snow and the wind picked up. The roads quickly became slushy and very slippery. Each footstep was more difficult than the last and much of the course was uphill. It became increasingly challenging as my illiotibial band on my right leg became sore from the extra strain and effort my legs were incurring. I was running against the wind. My face and eyelashes were coated in ice. I had to squint to protect my eyes. Fortunately, I'd taken Allan's advice and wore my waterproof wind breaker; it ended up keeping me dry.

After the first five kilometers, I didn't think I would be able to complete the run. Then I began some positive self-talk to get through that mental wall: Persist and persevere. It worked. I pushed myself, telling myself to lift my feet one at a time. My strides were short to deal with the slippery roads. My pace was slower than usual. I couldn't sprint to the finish line as I'd done in past races. My time was 1:13:53. Ten minutes off my last 10 km race, but I was pleased to be under 75 minutes. The winter conditions had made the run very challenging. I felt relieved when the race was over. I was so happy to finish. My goal was just to complete this crazy race. And that I did. Plus, I got my finisher's medal!

The first day of March signalled a new day, a new month, and time for some new challenges. I registered online for the Ottawa Race Weekend half marathon that would take place in late May. As soon as I completed my registration and clicked Enter to finalize my payment, I felt committed and excited. Spring was coming and soon I'd be back in training mode. I wanted to work on speed, so I started doing fartleks on the treadmill, alternating my pace between walking at 3.5 mph and running at 6.5 mph. I knew I had to push myself harder if I wanted to improve.

By late April, I realized there was just a month to go before the Ottawa Race Weekend. Time for a mental recalibration. I started running some longer distances to prepare for the half marathon. I needed to get in one long run, one short run, and one medium run per week, increasing my weekly mileage.

"Why did I sign up for this race?" I asked myself. I remembered the exhilaration of crossing the finish line after my first half marathon the previous fall. What an accomplishment it had been for this former couch potato. I wanted to experience that thrill again. I laced up my shoes and hit the pavement.

Before I knew it, it was late May and race day was here. My friend and fellow runner Paula and I arrived about an hour before the race. We stopped to use the washrooms in a hotel but decided to make one last pit stop 20 minutes before gun time; however, by that time there were hundreds of people lined up at the porta potties. We figured it was just nerves and that we really didn't have to go to the washroom.

There were over 10,000 runners in this event and many more thousands of spectators. The streets were jam packed. Paula and I had different estimated completion times. Mine was between 2 hours and 15 minutes and 2 hours and 30 minutes. We wished each other good luck and headed to our corresponding corrals. The elite runners were situated at the very front of the pack. There were barriers on either side of the street to keep the spectators off of the course. I was worried that when the race started, people would push the barriers and a crush would ensue. Fortunately, everyone was calm and polite, walking slowly around the barriers or climbing over them without any pushing. I climbed over a barrier and started walking with the crowd of runners towards the start line. We each had a timing chip on our shoe. Our individual time counters didn't kick in until we stepped over the start line, so it didn't matter if it took a few minutes to get there.

My heart pounded with anticipation as I stepped over the start line and began a slow run shoulder to shoulder with thousands of fellow runners. After a few blocks, the crowd thinned out and I picked up speed. The first two kilometers went amazingly well. I did that portion averaging five and a half minutes per kilometer, which was extremely fast for me.

By the fourth kilometer, all I could think about was the urge to pee. Since I was hoping to get a new personal best at this race, I didn't want to waste precious minutes waiting for a porta potty like I did in the Canada Army Run. After several minutes of contemplating my situation, I did what real runners do—I ran behind a cluster of bushes, pulled down my pants, and had a quick pee. I closed my eyes, figuring that if I couldn't see anyone, no one could see me. I was done in a flash and quickly rejoined the race.

My first 10 kilometers felt great. I don't think I ever had such a good 10K. The route took us from Ottawa, Ontario into Hull, Quebec which has lots of elevation. Every time I thought we were done running up what I hoped would be the last thigh-burning hill, there was another one right around the corner.

The second half of the run took us back into Ottawa which was flatter and easier, but I began to feel a bit fatigued and I could tell I was slowing down. By the 14th kilometer, I was feeling the heat. I didn't want to drink a lot, just a few sips of water at each water station. I didn't realize at the time that I was getting dehydrated. As I got to 17th then 18th kilometer, I started feeling light-headed. I was getting carb depleted and quickly running out of energy. By the 19th kilometer, I seriously questioned whether I'd be able to finish. I made up my mind right there and then that I was not going to give up, not after coming this far. I saw quite a few runners who by now were walking. I even saw a few runners down, being tended to by first-aid responders. But I struggled along, forcing myself to put one foot in front of the other.

Spectators cheered us on. (I love running races because it's the only time when people cheer for me!) Various bands played music. People held up signs. I looked around for my own cheering squad. I eventually saw Allan, Jesse, and Joshua cheering. I literally couldn't afford to waste any energy shouting out to them; instead, I clapped my hands to get their attention, then I passed by them, and had a quick look back and a wave before continuing on. That was the only time during the entire race that I looked back; I didn't want to see how many (or how few) runners were behind me. I wanted to focus on where I was headed.

Towards the end, people were cheering and shouting, "You're almost there!" but there was still one kilometer to go. It seemed like a huge distance although I knew it was not. Then I saw the sign for 750 meters, then 500, then 400, and then 300. Each 100 meters was a mini victory. My legs were aching. I was exhausted. I thought I might faint. I didn't have any remaining energy to sprint towards the finish line. I felt like I was trying to sprint, but my body wouldn't cooperate.

I saw Allan, Jesse, and Joshua again just before I crossed the finish line. Finishing was a moment of both joy and relief. I eyed a medic standing next to a wheelchair. My legs felt like rubber. I was unstable on my feet. I had the urge to head in that direction and ask for medical attention. Instead, I kept on walking. A volunteer removed the timing chip from my shoe and I had to walk another few meters to get my medal. What a walk. I didn't know if I'd make it. Someone put a medal around my neck and instructed me to head to the athletes-only area. I had to wait in line for a couple of minutes to get a bottle of water, a bagel, a banana, and some much needed slices of orange. I was starving and thirsty. I gobbled the oranges as I needed sugar to combat my dizziness. I ate voraciously, chomping on the bagel. It was so good. I went to lie down on a grassy area and put my legs up against a tree. Finally, I picked up my checked baggage and phoned Allan. We met up and took some photos with my medal and then we got ice cream. I was still feeling weak, unlike the energetic ending I had at the Canada Army Run. We drove home and I had a hot, relaxing bath and a rest.

I didn't urinate much for almost 12 hours. I was dehydrated. I checked my blood pressure and it was too low. I drank juice and lots of water that day and by evening I was better. It would take many races before I finally figured out the right amount of carbs and fluids to consume in order to prevent dehydration, electrolyte imbalance, and low blood sugar. Each person's body reacts differently. I've seen people faint and collapse during and after races. Fortunately, that hasn't happened to me.

My calves were sore for two days, making it difficult to walk down the stairs. I posted my results on Facebook and received many congratulatory messages from friends. It felt good to achieve my goal. My chip time was 2 hours 31 minutes and 47 seconds, a full minute and 20 seconds better than my Army Run time. It was my new personal best!

Towards the end of the race, I remember telling myself I will never do this again; it's too hard. What's the point? By the next day, I was already googling to find some new races in the vicinity and I was looking forward to September's Canada Army Run. Running a race is like giving birth—the pain and suffering is quickly forgotten as you focus on the joyfulness of the outcome.

I remember kissing my medal after it was placed around my neck. I'd worked hard for it. I hung it up in my basement home gym on my wall of fame, next to my other medals. My bulletin board was getting filled up with medals and race number bibs. Either I'd have to stop racing or get a second bulletin board. Hmmm, I wondered what I'd do about that.

Personal Best Practices

o   Be fearless.

o   It's never too late to try something new.

o   Live each day to the fullest.

o   Make time to do the things you enjoy.

o   You can inspire others with your actions.

o   You are more powerful than you know.

o   You are your most important competitor.

o   Live like a warrior, not like a worrier.

o   Push yourself.

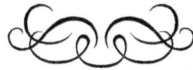

9 EVALUATION

I was going for it no matter what!

It was now the end of June, 2009. I realized it was exactly one year ago that I'd started my exercise log on my laptop. Every day I had diligently logged, at a general level, what exercise I did. What started as a summer project to motivate myself while I was at my cottage and away from my gym had morphed into an ongoing obsession. I felt compelled to record my daily exercise. I reviewed my log and extracted summary statistics for the year. What can I say? I like numbers. I'd run 607 kilometers including two half marathons and two 10 kilometer races; I'd done 146 one-hour workouts on my own; I'd participated in 32 strength classes and 33 kickboxing classes; I'd gone to 21 yoga classes; I'd walked on the treadmill 52 times for different lengths of times, at different speeds and inclines; and I'd gone rollerblading 11 times. I'd had 55 days of inactivity during the year, which equates to 15 percent of inactive days, or an average of one day off per week. That may seem incredible to some people. To others, it may seem rather ordinary. I take the approach of comparing myself to my own past performance, and not to other people's performances or expectations. I was impressed with my progress especially considering I'd been sedentary until just a couple of years earlier.

I had completed a year in which I'd dedicated myself mentally and physically to fitness and to self-improvement. Now that the year was over, was my journey complete? No! Time to start a new log file and start recording all over again; more importantly, time to reflect on how far I'd come and where I wanted to go in the coming months and year. Time to evaluate, to take a moment to pat myself on the back for a great year, and to assess what I wanted to do next. Where did I want to be one year from now? Would continuing on this same path get me to a new destination? Probably not. I wasn't satisfied with the notion of simply maintaining the same level of fitness. I wanted to come up with some new challenges and goals for myself.

Again, I'd been noticing that my eating habits were not nearly as healthy as I wanted. I was pleased with myself for having kicked my soft drink habit six months earlier on January 1, 2009. I also hadn't eaten at fast-food restaurants all year. These were two major lifestyle changes that I was able to maintain without a problem—and I continue to maintain them to this day. Yet, I was still often indulging in unhealthy treats.

I became more aware of my lack of self-control—a lifelong struggle—when I made my son Joshua a birthday party. He wanted lots of junk food so I gave in. He and his little friends watched a movie at our home while pigging out on chips. Pizza was followed by make-your-own sundaes with all the toppings. There were a couple of leftover jumbo bags of chips after the party. I put them away in a cupboard. What I should have done was throw them in the garbage. My old nemesis, whom I refer to as Chips, surfaced from the recesses of my mind. Chips called me to that cupboard and urged me to rip open a bag.

"I'll just have a handful," I told myself, but of course that didn't happen. I had several handfuls, then a large bowlful. Before I knew it, I'd eaten half of the jumbo bag. Over the next couple of days, my inner glutton kept resurfacing, like one of Sybil's multiple personalities. It wasn't the real me—or was it?! It wasn't the me that I wanted to be! It was the old me acting in my old ways. Bad habits are hard to crush. Addiction is a more appropriate term. I often hear people say things like, "I'm a recovering alcoholic. I've been in recovery for 10 years." Food can have the same addictive power.

Addictions never truly die. They hide within us and lurk, waiting to surface in a moment of weakness. Food-related addictions are similar. It's so easy to fall off the wagon. With all the excess junk food in my house, I gorged on chips until there were none left. I felt disgusted with myself. For the next few weeks, I kept reminding myself to eat healthy foods, but I craved treats more than ever. Once you fall off the wagon, it's hard to get back on. I had a more difficult time passing by the chocolate bars and chips next to the grocery store cash register. I started allowing myself more treats here and there. I knew then that my new and perhaps most important goal for the coming months would be to clean up my eating habits. I had to employ some new strategies to get back into maintenance mode.

I bought *The Eat-Clean Diet* book by Tosca Reno (2006). I had read about Tosca on the internet. Here was a beautiful, fit, lean, and muscular 50-year-old woman who had previously been extremely overweight and out of shape. She lost a lot of weight and made a career out of teaching others how to eat better. She also changed her sedentary lifestyle and became extremely fit through exercise, even participating in female bodybuilding competitions.

Many of her tips were common sense, but perhaps things I'd let slide or forgotten about. This was just-in-time information that I needed at that point. Some of the tips that jumped out at me were reminders to eat lots of fruits and vegetables and lean protein, to stay away from processed foods and simple carbohydrates, and to put more thought and effort into my daily food planning and preparation. She also reinforced the idea of eating five or six small meals per day rather than three large ones, so that you feel satiated and in control instead of stuffed or famished.

I wanted to eat clean in July and August. Allan and our children pretty much ate whatever I put in the fridge, so if I provided healthier options, they'd eat them. It would be a big challenge for my younger son Joshua. He was still a very picky eater. Introducing small changes over time would be the strategy I'd have to use with him. For example, the day after I read Tosca's book, I saw Joshua holding a huge slab of sour dough bread. This simple carbohydrate was not a healthy choice. I suggested to Joshua that I make him a fruit plate. I never asked him to put the bread away. I cut a Golden Delicious apple into very thin slices so they looked like chips. I cut up a few luscious strawberries and laid the fruit out on a small plate. Joshua's eyes widened with delight. He asked if he could put the bread away and have the fruit instead. I was thrilled. I told him that I'd read that people who eat lots of fresh fruits and veggies live healthier and longer lives. I didn't say anything else as I didn't want to harp on the issue, especially since he was happy to eat the fruit.

Over the coming weeks and months, I'd try to make similar suggestions for better choices. Hopefully, Allan and Jesse would buy into this healthier way of eating, too. I wanted to reduce my daily bread servings—something that had always been a struggle for me since I loved bread. Because of my chronic kidney disease, for nearly 20 years I've had to limit my protein intake. I eat less protein than average people. When you exercise, you need more protein to rebuild your muscles. I was exercising and getting stronger but not able to increase my protein intake accordingly. Consuming a limited amount of protein left me feeling hungry much of the time, so I turned to carbohydrates to feel satiated. My dietary restrictions will always pose an added challenge for me to stay strong and fit and at the same time, keep off excess weight.

I also wanted to try to have more vegetarian meals. For health reasons, I'd already been limiting the amount of red meat that I ate and served my family. However, I'd previously included cheese in many vegetarian meals, such as lasagna. Cheese is high in sodium, which is especially bad for people with a medical condition that requires them to keep their blood pressure low. Unlike in the past, when I'd given up and just ate everything, this time I put in the effort and faced my dietary challenges. I wanted to be more than fit; I wanted to optimize my health.

I was determined to be more organized and plan several days' worth of meals, rather than shop and eat spontaneously. I'd try to shop around meal plans.

Just as I embarked on this clean eating approach, I happened to come down with a terrible bout of stomach flu. At first I thought it was food poisoning that I'd contracted on a weekend trip to Toronto, but soon I heard that this bug was going around. I was violently ill all night with horrible cramps. I was exhausted the next day. I thought it was over and done with, but the cramps, nausea, and diarrhea hit me again for a couple of hours the next night. It felt like the episode I'd experienced the previous summer. This time, I barely ate solid food for three days other than toast and oatmeal. I kept myself hydrated with water mixed with some of the electrolyte replacement powder I had for running. Unfortunately, the bug struck me again later in the week and I spent the night either on the toilet or in a fetal position on the bathroom floor in agony. In hindsight, I should have been hospitalized.

Finally, by week's end the bug was gone for good. I weighed myself and discovered that I was down to 129 pounds. I hadn't weighed that little in at least 15 years. I felt weak and too thin. For the first time in 20 years, I wanted to gain weight. I made pasta and meatballs and had a moderate portion that I chased with a protein bar for extra calories. I even ate a big ice cream cone the next day at the mall. Within a couple of days of generous eating, I was up to 132 pounds and felt terrific. That's how much I weighed nine months prior, just at the end of the previous summer.

⁂

Because of the stomach virus, I hadn't exercised in almost a week and was not feeling motivated. I was actually enjoying not exercising. The longest I'd gone in the past year without some form of exercise was two days. I knew I had to get started. I got back into hill running near my cottage. The first time I went out, I had to walk a few times going up some of the hills. There were lots of biting insects but that didn't deter me. I wore my trusty bug net over my entire head. It was hot under that thing but it kept the bugs from eating my face. A few tough hill runs and I was feeling strong once again.

The July weather was quite disappointing, with rain many days, so it was hard to get out kayaking or running. Whenever the clouds parted and it cleared up, I took advantage and went for a run. Now it was mid-July and with just over two months to go until the Canada Army Run, I knew I had to start getting in some long runs. I couldn't do that at the cottage since it was too hilly. I'd have to start making trips to the city to fit those in.

In search of inspiration, I borrowed some running books from the public library. *Ultra Marathon Man: Confessions of an All-Night Runner* by Dean Karnazes was interesting and motivating. This autobiography was about running some of the longest, most gruelling endurance races under the most difficult conditions, from the brutal heat of the desert to the unbearable cold of the Antarctic.

One quote that particularly resonated with me was, "If it comes easy, it doesn't require extraordinary effort, you're not pushing hard enough: It's supposed to hurt like hell" (p. 23). Karnazes lives by these words that came from his junior high school running coach.

Well, I've never voluntarily done anything that hurt like hell. My gastrointestinal cramps had hurt like hell but they were not voluntary. My half marathons had not hurt like hell, but they'd been big challenges that pushed me beyond my previously self-constructed mental and physical limits. Karnazes' book and the quote in particular reinforced my mantra to persist and persevere. In any future races or other challenges, I would try to remember the essence of that quote. I would try to push myself and improve on my personal best. I was not competing against anyone other than myself. I wanted to keep pushing myself to get just that much better, that much stronger, that much faster.

Jesse and Joshua went to summer camp in late July. They would be gone for almost a month so Allan and I booked a trip for ourselves. We'd fly to Seattle where we'd spend a few days sightseeing and from there we'd take a one-week Alaskan cruise. Friends had told me that Alaska was cool and rainy so I packed a fleece vest, several hoodies, a sweater, gloves, a hat, even the wicking long johns and shirt that I'd worn as an under layer on our heli-hiking trip the previous summer. I also packed lots of shorts and T-shirts because I planned on using the gym facilities at the hotel and on the ship. Having been on a couple of cruises, I knew that I'd have to exercise during my vacation to burn off some of the extra calories I'd surely consume.

Seattle in late July was unusually hot. We were on the cusp of a heat wave which was great since summer in Ottawa had, thus far, been rainy and disappointing. Allan found out that there was going to be a big running event in Seattle during our time there. The races would be followed by the Seattle Torchlight Fair parade consisting of floats covered in lights and people dressed up as pirates. There was a 5 km and an 8 km race. He suggested we do the 5K, but I told him I thought that would be too easy for him. He'd been doing a bit of running out at our cottage. I was confident he could manage a fairly flat 8 km run. He agreed, perhaps with a bit of coaxing from me. We registered the day before the event. The run would begin at 6:30 p.m.

I expected it to be warm but comfortable at that time of day.

On the morning of the race, hundreds of people were already setting up chairs and jockeying for good viewing positions along the parade route. I'd never seen such enthusiasm. Spectators had coolers filled with food and drinks, and board games to help pass the many hours as they awaited the parade.

Prior to the race, I prepared two bottles of electrolyte replenishment drink for Allan and myself. I advised him to carry his bottle during the race and take a few sips every few minutes. He was skeptical and felt he wouldn't need to carry a drink for a short run. He thought he could rely on the drinking stations. I insisted, so he reluctantly took the bottle. We headed off to the Qwest Stadium which was the starting point.

I felt excited as I saw other runners arriving for the races. There were thousands of registered participants. I told Allan not to stick with me during the run because I was much slower than him. I wanted him to have a good finishing time and not be held back by me. We agreed on a meeting place to find each other after the race. I was psyched up and ready to go.

The race began and we were off. Just a few seconds into the race, I saw Allan fall flat on the ground. I didn't know at the time that someone had accidentally tripped him. I stopped and ask him if he was okay. He was a real trouper; he got up, his knee and hands scraped and bleeding, and kept on running. That was the last I saw of him until after the race.

The course included an uphill portion along a viaduct. It was difficult and it was warmer than I'd anticipated. I sipped from my bottle every few minutes and that helped. It was fun to be running in a different city. Around the 4th or 5th kilometer, I started to feel like I was breathing hard and my heart was pounding rapidly. I tried to focus more and relax. For a moment, I asked myself why I was doing this, but then I got that negative thought out of my head. Eventually we were all running along the road where the parade would be, so thousands of people were there to cheer all of us on. That gave me the motivation to keep on going.

I wasn't familiar with the city or the route, so every time I came around a corner I thought I was near the finish line. The last part of the run was downhill and that's where I felt a surge of energy. I began running faster and felt very comfortable. Then I saw the finish line and I felt so strong and energized that I was able to sprint at full speed to the end. I don't think I have ever had such a strong finish. I felt terrific. This event had no finishers' medals which was disappointing because I love to collect medals. Nonetheless, I was happy to have participated.

I went over to the food table and sucked on some orange quarters and wolfed down a bagel and a drink. I meandered through the throngs of finishers and looked at the various vendors' kiosks, then headed over to the corner where I was supposed to meet Allan. Sure enough he was there. He had finished and he'd come in ahead of me as I expected. I was happy to see him, but he looked dazed and confused. I had him sit on the curb and I told him that his eyes were bugging out. He said I'd have to drive home since he was dizzy. Well, I knew then that something was wrong because we had come to Seattle on an airplane, not by car. I told him to stay put and I got him a bottle of electrolyte drink from a kiosk. He chugged it down but when he stood up, he nearly toppled over. I got some medics to take a look at him. They asked if he was diabetic, which he is not. They decided he needed fluids, so we went into the ambulance where they administered a bag of fluid intravenously. They asked if he wanted to go to the hospital or return to the hotel. We agreed to play it safe and had them take us to the nearby Swedish Hospital. We had excellent service. No one asked us for identification or a credit card upfront even though we were foreigners. Allan was taken immediately into Emergency and given an EKG, blood tests, and two more bags of fluid. Fortunately, after a couple of hours he was fine, his heart rate was normal again, and his blood test was fine.

We took a taxi back to the hotel. I picked up some food from a nearby restaurant and we ate in our room. He felt perfectly fine and felt a bit silly for having gone to the hospital, but I think it's good we went since we were heading off on our cruise the following morning. From this experience, Allan gained an appreciation for staying hydrated—and for listening to his wife!

⚜

The next morning we headed off on our cruise. It was a lovely week. We had four ports-of-call: Ketchikan, Juneau, Skagway, and then Victoria, British Columbia. Allan was determined to do active excursions; so, despite my reluctance, we went ziplining in Ketchikan. I found the first two ziplines scary. I felt myself free fall as soon as I jumped off the ledge. I hate that feeling. I closed my eyes, gritted my teeth, and held on for dear life, praying for it to end. Within a few seconds I was zipping upwards to the other end of the rope and I was enjoying the ride. The last six ziplines were more horizontal, so I didn't feel any falling motion and I enjoyed the adventure. There were also a few rope challenges, such as crossing a shaky rope bridge.

In Juneau, it was my turn to choose an activity. I chose whale watching. We hadn't done that since our honeymoon many years earlier in Cape Cod. Watching majestic whales jump out of the icy water was breathtaking.

In Skagway, Allan insisted we not take the typical old-fashioned train ride that all the tourists take up the mountain and back. Instead, he managed to convince me to go up the mountain with a small group in a van, and we cycled down from 3200 feet. It seemed very scary to me since it was all downhill on a highway with cars and trucks whizzing by. I said I would hang out at the back of the pack and that he should go ahead, but within minutes I had made my way up towards the front and I wasn't scared at all. Sometimes, it's good to have a push and do something different. I never would have imagined cycling down a mountain in Alaska!

❦

Much of the focus of the cruise was the food. I tried to eat reasonably, but there were lots of temptations. There was a fresh cookie and cappuccino bar on the same deck as our cabin, so I had a couple of large, hot peanut butter or chocolate chip cookies every day for a snack. I ate moderate breakfasts, but definitely more calories than I would consume for breakfast at home. The lunch buffet offered an incredible array of choices. I couldn't help but notice the high number of obese passengers on the cruise. They really got good value for their money. The buffet offered two sizes of plates: a round dinner plate or an oval double-size plate. I always used the regular plate, but many people used the double-size plate and piled it high with mountains of food. Surprisingly, the portion sizes at the sit-down dinner restaurant were modest. I find most American restaurants give disgustingly huge portions. Luckily for my waistline, I

124

didn't like some of the desserts. My joke that week was that I had to have my pre-snack snack. There was all-day pizza, hamburgers, fries, and ice cream just in case someone was hungry between buffets and sit-down meals. I don't think there was a minute during the cruise when food was unavailable. Even when we went to our cabin late at night, there was a chocolate truffle waiting for each of us on our pillow. Of course I ate it!

When I got home, I weighed myself with trepidation. I only gained two pounds which is what I had considered a best-case scenario given all my extra snacks, desserts, and multi-course dinners. Phew! As soon as I got back to healthy eating, the extra pounds came off.

In August 2009, Allan and I celebrated our 18th wedding anniversary. Where did the years go? Our boys were still away at camp. Allan and I wanted to go out and celebrate, but I wasn't in the mood for a gourmet dinner. I suggested we go for a run together, but it was really hot that day. We decided to go for a bike ride. We cycled along the paths next to the Ottawa River. It was muggy and a light rain shower came down on us for a few minutes, but we kept on going until we cycled to the Byward Market area. We parked our bikes and went into a Mexican eatery for a very casual supper.

I had helmet hair from my bike helmet, and we were both sweaty and splattered with mud. The past 17 anniversaries had been at fancy restaurants and we'd been well-attired and neatly groomed. This was different. I was different. Allan was different, too. He'd been adopting more of a fitness lifestyle, though it was still a challenge for him to find time to exercise—or make time—because of his long work hours. That day, he'd finished work at 2 p.m. so we could spend time together. I really liked that. What a great gift. I didn't need more jewellery, flowers, or perfume. Spending time together doing something fun was just perfect. During dinner, a former colleague of mine recognized me as she walked by the restaurant patio pushing her baby in a stroller. She called my name and I came over and hugged her.

"Gloria, you look amazing. You're so slim. Not that you were ever fat!" she exclaimed. I hadn't seen her in three years but we had communicated via Facebook a few times. She looked slim as always even though her baby was just a few months old. I complimented her, we exchanged a few pleasantries, and then I had to excuse myself to rejoin Allan for our dinner. It was kind of cool that my old friend recognized me even though I'd changed. I later went to use the restroom and was appalled at how sweaty and sloppy I looked! No makeup, messy hair, muddy tank top. I never looked like that when she and I worked together. Athletes, I suppose, are more concerned with their fitness than their appearance. And of course, I was an athlete.

⚜

I saw my cottage neighbour Marie in mid-August and she proudly announced to me that she had registered for the Canada Army Run half marathon. I was so excited for her. She expressed some self-doubts, just as I'd done when I had registered for this event the year before. I knew Marie could do it. She was a regular runner and she told me she'd been training for longer runs with a group. Her most recent long run was 16 kilometers. I reassured her that if she could run that far, then 21.1 was not much of a stretch.

As we talked, I happened to have in my hand a book that I'd been reading called *The Five Secrets You Must Discover Before You Die* (2008).

"What are the secrets?" enquired Marie. I told her she'd have to read the book to find out. I smirked and then I decided to divulge one of the secrets that I thought would encourage her with her running goal.

"According to the seniors surveyed by the author, as you reach the end of your life, however long that is, what many people regret are not the risks they took, but the ones they didn't take because they were afraid. If you take risks, either you succeed or fail. The people the author interviewed typically felt that regardless of the outcome, the fact that they'd taken a risk was an accomplishment because they learned from their experience. If they didn't try something because of their fear of failure, they often regretted it later in life. Marie, you can apply this secret to your goal. Don't be afraid to try the half marathon. Think of the best-case scenario: You finish the run, get your medal, and feel an amazing sense of accomplishment that you carry in your heart for the rest of your life. Now think of the worse-case scenario: You're unable to finish for whatever reason. Maybe you are just too tired, or you get an injury, or you don't drink enough and get dehydrated. Whatever happens, you'll know that you tried your best and you'll learn from the experience. There's no shame in that. If you never try, you'll never know."

Marie smiled. Her eyes glistened.

"You know," she said, "I'm doing this because you encouraged me to go for it."

I had planted the seed, the little kernel of an idea in her head months ago. Yes, that was true. But she was the one who took that idea and ran with it, no pun intended. She was the one acting upon the idea, just as I'd done the year before. She had the courage to push past her fear of failure and train for something that would potentially become one of her greatest accomplishments.

"I'll see you at the finish line Marie," I told her with confidence. "And you'll get a cool army tag style medal that you can wear for a few days and show to your friends. You'll earn bragging rights when you cross that finish line, and your friends will be impressed because you're going to do something you've never done before and something that some of them may never do. It will be a real achievement and you'll feel incredible." And I felt incredible at that moment—me, an ordinary person doing an extraordinary thing— motivating and inspiring a friend to reach beyond what she'd previously thought were her limits.

❦

Before I knew it, the Canada Army Run was just one week away. I was trained and I was excited. My goal was to have a new personal best of less than 2 hours and 30 minutes. If I couldn't do that, I would definitely finish the entire run without stopping, as I'd done in my last two half marathons—pee stops excluded.

Just four days before the race, I got a frightening phone call. I'd had a breast MRI the week before, at my request due to my family history of breast cancer. The test suggested an abnormality and it was deemed necessary for me to have a breast biopsy as a follow-up. I was in shock. I was just thinking the other day how great I felt and how I was looking forward to the run. I cried. The specialist who'd

127

sent me for the MRI was on vacation. Fortunately, I was able to speak with my family doctor on the phone. She was very helpful. I had the MRI results faxed to her and she interpreted them for me. I asked her what she thought the chance was that I did have cancer. She said 50/50. That sounded pretty grim to me.

I was given an appointment for an ultrasound-guided biopsy on the 28th of September. I kept telling myself to wipe away the tears and not to get carried away imagining the worst. Many MRIs give false positives. I hoped this would be the case. I was filled with anxiety. I didn't want to alarm my sons so I didn't tell them anything and I put on a happy face in front of them.

This was a test. Would I be able to have the courage to get through the days ahead? Could I force myself to have a hopeful outlook? I made an electronic note in my new smart phone. It read, "No fear." It's easy for me to say that with respect to trying new fitness activities, but it wasn't so easy in light of this medical crisis. I'd have to try hard not to spend every waking moment thinking bad thoughts. I would do my run on the weekend and I'd give it my all. I wanted to be able to apply my warrior attitude to this scary situation and I tried to remain hopeful that the biopsy would be negative. There was nothing else I could do except wait.

The weather for the Canada Army Run was ideal. Clear, sunny skies with a cool start. Halfway through, it got rather warm. I wore a backpack style fluid carrier containing 1.5 litres of water mixed with electrolyte powder. I forced myself to sip every few minutes to prevent dehydration. I had a great pace during the first half and kept up with the 2 hour 20 minutes pace bunny. However, I slowed down during the second half. I felt good the entire time other than fatigue in my biceps and triceps. I got a bit light-headed in the last third of the race, but frequent sips of my beverage kept me going.

Throughout the race I tried to keep my mind off of my upcoming biopsy. I periodically had to distract myself and force my mind to focus on other things. I sang the lyric, "This train is bound for glory" over and over in my head. I must have sung it hundreds of times. It helped me re-focus whenever my mind started to wander into negative territory.

I remember seeing a heavy man running just ahead of me. The following caption was on the back of his T-shirt, "I may have a fat ass but I'm in front of you." Hilarious! Lots of the race was a blur as I pushed myself physically and mentally. As I approached the 20 km mark, I realized I only had a few short minutes to meet my goal of finishing in less than 2 hours and 30 minutes.

I summoned all of my remaining energy and picked up my pace. Photos of me that Allan would later show me revealed an intense look of determination on my face. I was grimacing. I was feeling a bit asthmatic. I was going for it no matter what! Nothing was going to stop me! As I saw the finish line, I ran with even more tenacity. I saw Allan, Jesse, and Joshua on the sidelines just meters from the finish line, cheering me on. This was it. I was going to do it. I sprinted across the finish line, raising my arms in triumph and nearly bursting into tears.

"Keep walking," directed the volunteers. Had they not instructed us to do that I think I would have collapsed right there. I kept walking and a young woman placed a medal around my neck. I kissed my medal. I had done it! I later found out my official time was 2 hours, 29 minutes, 11 seconds. I'd achieved my goal and another personal best on my third half marathon. What a feeling of euphoria!

Allan and the boys met me in the recovery area where I was lying on the ground on my back with my legs propped up against a tree. I phoned Marie to see how she'd done. She finished in just over 2 hours. Amazing! After a short rest and some food and water, Allan, the kids and I went home. I soaked in a hot bath then had a nap. I felt great except for a bit of generalized soreness. Only one small blister, no injuries. I was pleased. While it was not as exciting as my first run one year ago, it still felt great. It was still a solid challenge. Next, I had to get through my upcoming medical challenge and come out of it victorious—one way or another.

After two weeks that filled me with tremendous anxiety, I finally had my appointment in late September for an ultrasound-guided biopsy. The radiologist could not locate the lesion on the ultrasound, so the biopsy could not be performed. I was informed that I'd need to go for an MRI-guided biopsy instead. After waiting a few days and making several frantic phone calls to find out when my appointment would be, I found out it would be nearly two more weeks away. Such is the Canadian medical system.

Allan—who is a pathologist—obtained a copy of my original MRI report that identified my lesion as a lower risk category, which differed from my family doctor's interpretation of it being a 50 percent chance of cancer. Nonetheless, I was so overwhelmed with anxiety that I couldn't think logically. I was terrified that I'd be one of the unlucky ones to have a bad outcome. There was nothing to do but wait for the biopsy appointment. I tried to use positive self-talk, to remain focused on good thoughts, to do enjoyable activities, and to keep myself busy and my mind occupied.

Only Allan knew what I was going through. I didn't want to frighten our children. I didn't have the courage to tell anyone else. Lynne could tell something was wrong when I didn't come to the gym for a few days. She asked what was going on. When she pushed the issue, I got irritated and told her not to be so nosy. It was my defense mechanism. I knew I'd burst into tears if I shared what I was going through. I wanted to keep it together as much as possible. I felt like I was emotionally spiralling out of control. I thought that if I confided in a few friends, they would keep asking me the status. With the medical delays and all the waiting, I just didn't want to discuss it. I also didn't want my family to worry, especially my elderly father.

If one of my close friends or a relative were going through such an anxious time, I would hope they would confide in me and that I would be able to be there for them. For better or for worse, I'm a very private person. So private, in fact, that the thought of publishing this book and divulging the personal details of my journey—my medical problems in particular—caused me great angst. After much contemplation and introspection, I felt the importance of my story and the potential for it to help other people far outweighed my desire for privacy.

I continued to wait for my MRI appointment date. I hoped that the day would soon come when I could tell some friends and family members what I had gone through and that the biopsy had turned out to be negative. I prayed that this would happen. I just had to hang tight and wait it out. When I didn't think about the possible diagnosis of cancer—which of course made me think of the living hell my late mother had gone through—I felt just fine.

One day when I was down in my basement, I came across a photo of Allan, the boys, and me from about three years earlier when we were on a family vacation. Man, I was overweight then! That must have been at my peak weight of 157 or close to it. My face looked bloated, my bust was bigger, my arms were flabby, and I was thick around the middle.

One of my cousins had recently referred to me as the Super Jock, but I still had difficulty consistently thinking of myself as athletic. What would it take to change my mindset? I sometimes felt as though I'd been fooled into believing that I was athletic. I felt like the emperor in the fable *The Emperor's New Clothes* who'd been led to believe he was dressed in royal clothing when he was actually naked. Could everyone see a different truth from my own? Was I unknowingly a fool? Other times, I really did feel that I was a runner, that I was invincible, and that I was fearless.

It's funny how we can have different perceptions of ourselves compared to how others perceive us. People were telling me that I looked amazingly fit and lean, yet sometimes I remained fixated on my flaws. It's like looking at a Rembrandt painting and seeing one imperfect brush stroke rather than enjoying and appreciating the masterpiece. I continued to remind myself to think differently and to consistently, not intermittently, see myself in a positive light. In terms of giving positive strokes, I needed to learn to be as generous with myself as I was with others.

And then, after this self-analysis, I felt foolish for even thinking about such trivial matters as appearance when I was a week away from that dreaded biopsy. Who knows what life has in store for us or what awaits us just around the corner? I promised myself that if the outcome of the biopsy left me physically unscathed—if I did not have cancer—I would never again put myself down for my appearance. But then I immediately modified that promise and told myself that no matter the outcome, I would never put myself down again. Only positive thoughts and high self-esteem. That would be a good challenge.

I don't know how I hung on for 28 days waiting for the biopsy. And more incredibly, I don't know how I made it through the biopsy procedure. I'm the world's worst patient. I had to lie face down. I closed my eyes and felt myself being slid into the MRI machine. I felt panic-stricken. I'd developed claustrophobia a few years earlier in the same type of machine during some kidney imaging tests. I wanted to press the panic button and scream, "Get me out of here!" Instead, I visualized myself running and feeling free with the wind in my hair. I imagined running the last portion of a half marathon, seeing the finish line in the distance, feeling the sense of achievement. I reminded myself over and over that I am a warrior. The visualization and the positive self-talk got me through that scary biopsy. As the radiologist, the resident, and technical assistants performed their tasks and chatted to one another, I tried to remain focused on running. As the radiologist instructed the resident to insert the needle to get the tissue samples from within my breast, I imagined myself running on a beach. I pretended that the air circulating inside the MRI machine was a gentle breeze. That's what kept me sane.

There was no physical pain, minimal discomfort. Fear was the enemy. I willed myself through it even when I could feel my arms shaking from nerves and my heart palpitating as I lay trapped in the machine.

Once it was all over and I was allowed to leave the recovery area, only then as I walked with Allan through the parking lot and got to our car did I break down in tears. The stress, the worrying about the possible bad outcome, not the biopsy itself, is what freaked me out. "Please Lord" had become my new mantra. How many times I said that to myself in my mind, over and over, during those 28 days, I'll never know. I'd have to wait a few more days until the results of the biopsy would be ready and my doctor would contact me. The waiting was so stressful. Waiting. Waiting. Waiting. Like the longest race of my life that seemed to go on and on, the finish line so close and yet so far.

I had hoped to go to the gym the following day to get back into my routine and keep my mind busy. Time at home alone was not good at this point, but I had bleeding from the spot where the needle had been inserted. I packed my sports bra with a thick wad of gauze and kept rotating it to soak up the blood. No exercise for me for a few days. But I had the Mothers Against Drunk Drivers 10 km race to do in 5 days. I hoped that by then I'd have good news about my biopsy and that I'd have an amazingly joyful run.

I was totally dysfunctional on the morning that I was to receive my test results. I stayed in bed. I couldn't drive Joshua to school. When Allan told him that Mummy wasn't feeling well and that he'd drive him to school, I overheard Joshua remark that I was being lazy. If only he knew what I was going through. But I wanted to protect him and keep it to myself.

I'd been awake since 2:30 a.m., feeling mentally debilitated. I stayed in bed that morning, waiting anxiously for the phone to ring, waiting to hear my result. The plan was for Allan to speak with the pathologist—his colleague—who'd examined my biopsy. Then Allan would call me either way with the result.

Finally, the phone rang. I swear I saw a vision of a large truck speeding towards me. I felt it coming closer and closer and I shuddered as it was about to hit me head on. Then Allan told me everything was okay and my results were all negative. I did not have cancer! At first I thought he was just saying that so I wouldn't get upset. I had to ask him to repeat what he'd said as I couldn't quite absorb and process it. He repeated the good news and I burst out crying. The immense sense of relief flowed through my tears.

For weeks I had felt as though my life was on hold. Not knowing had been the hardest part. It was finally over.

❧❦❧

Life returned to normal. Now it was mid-October and it was the day of the MADD Dash race. I'd planned on running the 10K. Joshua would do the 5K walk/run escorted by Jesse. However, Jesse was not feeling well that morning, so I switched to the 5K and escorted Joshua. It was his first timed race. We put on our numbered bibs and timing chips.

When the race started, I grabbed his little hand and we bolted across the start line. I was surprised by how much running Joshua could do, especially since he was only nine years old. Initially, he had said he was only doing the race to get a medal. He wanted a medal because he'd seen how excited I was each time I received a medal. Once we got started, he kept running until he got winded and red in the face. I had to tell him to take walking breaks, then we'd run a bit

133

more. As we saw the finish line a hundred meters ahead of us, I once again grabbed his hand and we ran energetically as onlookers cheered. We sprinted across the finish line hand-in-hand. I was beaming with pride for my little Joshua. I had the honor of placing his very first medal around his neck and then we watched other runners finish their races. Given the scary situation I'd recently been through, I felt immense gratitude to be there with Joshua, sharing a special time together.

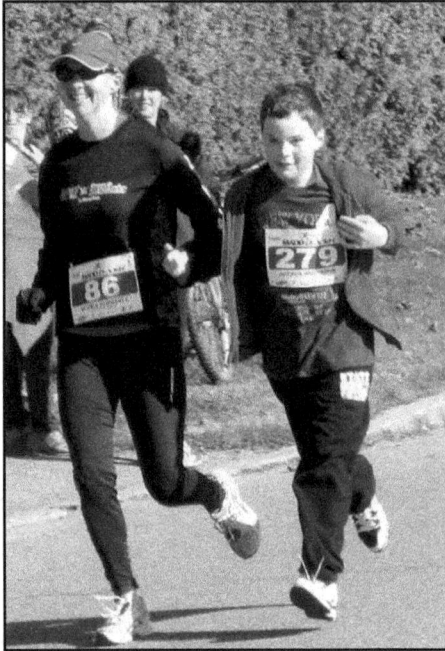

Experiencing Joshua's first race with him was pure joy for me on several levels.

In November, I proposed to the gym's manager that we have a running club. I would lead it. She agreed. It would start in January, 2010.

Meanwhile, I mustered the courage to borrow a personal trainer course manual from Lynne. Even though I didn't yet feel totally committed to taking the course—due, mainly to my fear of failure—I finally felt ready to examine the manual and see how complex the content was. From there, I could decide if I felt I could learn that kind of material. In retrospect, of course I was capable of learning that material. Any high school grad can take that course. I have a master's degree. I'm intelligent. But at that time, I was still plagued with some self-doubts.

As I read through the first few chapters, there was, indeed, a lot of information that was foreign to me, but also a lot of common-sense information. I toyed with the idea of writing the certification exam. I thought it was something I could do in the winter, not with the intention of using it to springboard into a new career, but to use it to grow as a person. I needed to start thinking about some new personal goals for 2010 and becoming a certified personal trainer was one thing that I was definitely considering adding to my list.

In mid-December, the running club was advertised in the community center winter catalog. A few women approached me to ask about the club. One said she'd like to learn to run 5 kilometers but she thought she was too old. I asked her how old she was and she said 47.

"I'll be 46 this month," I informed her. She looked very surprised. I suppose she thought I was younger than that. When I first started working out, I thought the trainers who were my age were much younger than me. In general, I think when you're in shape and feel energetic, you feel younger and exude a certain youthfulness. I explained to her what we'd be doing in the club and how I could work with her to build up her endurance. She seemed pleased.

❧

On December 31, 2009, I took a few moments to reflect back on the year. I realized that I have the power to control most aspects of my life. Yes, sometimes there are things beyond our control. When such events occur in our lives, we have to face them head on. I learned from my cancer scare that no matter what our circumstances, we can get through them and try our best to conquer them. I'd deteriorated into an emotional wreck when I waited for my biopsy results. I should have been more optimistic.

I've since read Dr. Wayne Dyer's book *You'll See it When You Believe It* (1989), which prompted me to try harder to use the power of my mind to overcome negative thoughts. I decided that in 2010, I would be more confident than ever about all aspects of myself and my life. Through conscious practice, I would train my brain to think in more productive ways.

2010 was going to be a great year. I was going to allow my mind to envelope itself in positive thoughts and simmer in a level of optimism that would become contagious. As I celebrated my birthday, I came up with my motto for how I felt: "I'm 46 and fabulous!"

Personal Best Practices

- o Take a moment to pat yourself on the back.
- o Have no regrets.
- o Think positive thoughts.
- o Keep challenging yourself.
- o Do away with self-limiting beliefs.
- o Share your enthusiasm—it's contagious.
- o You can choose some challenges. Some challenges choose you.
- o Practice gratitude by recognizing life's simple moments as special.
- o You're as old as you think you are.
- o Each race has a finish line.

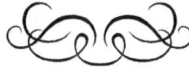

10 BELIEF

I have learned that I am capable of anything.

One of the early lines in this book was, "Let's think of getting fit as a project." When I started writing this book, I had recently exited the world of high tech, a world of projects containing timelines, plans, milestones, tasks, and resources. Getting fit is definitely a project; but for me it became so much more. It became a state of mind and a part of my being. Getting fit became more than eating well and exercising. Fitness is now my way of life.

When I started on my journey, I felt lost and insignificant because I no longer had a career. I felt depressed. I was plagued with anxiety and a sense of hopelessness about my medical situation.

Since then, my mindset has shifted. I've changed. My attitude has changed. The way that I think has changed. Through fitness, I have learned that I am capable of anything, even pushing myself physically and bursting through self-imposed, artificial barriers.

⸎

When I was a child, my family was not into sports. My parents did not participate in sports as adults or when they themselves were children. I have no recollection of my parents or brother watching sports on TV. Imagine a Canadian family that didn't watch hockey! I was a bit sporty as a child, but I never played competitive sports. I never tried out for teams. Academics were my focus when I was growing up. That was what my parents encouraged most. They wanted me to have a university education and career opportunities that they never had.

In my forties, I learned that what one does in their youth does not have to dictate or limit what they do at a different stage of life. What we experience, enjoy, or value at one point does not necessarily have to be what we pursue later. We are not fixed. We are fluid. We have the capacity to change and grow, to learn new skills, and gain new strengths. That's what makes life interesting.

When I was laid off, I initially felt sad about no longer working in high tech and I missed that feeling of self-worth that I'd always associated with having a career. It took some time but I have since come to realize that I am just as much of a contributor to my family and to society. It's just that now my contributions manifest in a different form. Many of the lifestyle changes that I adopted not only helped me, but they trickled down to, and benefited my family. Through personal training and eventually, through speaking engagements and writing, I would help many other people as well.

I now believed in myself in ways that I never could have imagined a short time ago. Talk about paradigm shift! I felt empowered. I felt strong and capable. I knew I could achieve whatever I set my mind to and invested my efforts in.

My late mother used to say, "God helps those who help themselves." She was right. I was helping myself, and in return, God was helping me.

Whether you believe in yourself, in a higher power, or both, what matters is that you believe. And if you believe, you will see the possibilities and discover a path to achieve your goals.

There comes a point in time when each of is faced with a fork in the road. To take the road less travelled is a risky endeavour but filled with new possibilities. To take the road with which we're already familiar is easier, more comfortable, and less stressful. Sometimes we need a change, a challenge, and a kind of stress that energizes us into action.

⤜⟲⟳⤛

It was the end of January 2010 when I stood at the fork in the road as I contemplated my choices. I could make up my mind that this would be the year I'd run a full marathon or I could do another half marathon. With just four months to go until Ottawa Race Weekend in May, I very soon had to decide because I'd need lots of training for a full marathon. Was I mentally prepared for this huge challenge? What would I get out of it? If I tried it and failed to finish, would I be disappointed or would I find joy in knowing that I gave it my best shot and conquered my fear of failure? If I went with the half marathon, which I knew I could finish because I'd already completed three of those, would I feel a great sense of accomplishment as I reached the finish line or would I be disappointed that I hadn't gone for what I thought was the ultimate physical goal? Did I really want to run a marathon or did I just want attention and respect from my peers? I asked myself what it was I was seeking. What would I get out of attempting a full marathon? Perhaps self-satisfaction. Perhaps the knowledge that once again I was doing something I could have never in my wildest dreams imagined doing. I wanted to do it once in my lifetime. I felt like this was the right time. It wouldn't get easier in the years ahead. I was at my peak fitness, so why not? 42.2 kilometers. What was there to lose?

⚮

At my next nephrology appointment, I asked my doctor whether it was medically safe for me to attempt a full marathon. He advised against it because such a long run—and all the practice runs leading up to it—cause muscle breakdown, which can damage the kidneys. Was I willing to risk further damage that could result in kidney failure? Since my kidney function was already significantly compromised, he felt I should stick to shorter distances, even less than half marathons. Based on this information, I reluctantly made the final decision that I would not train for a marathon. However, I would train for another half marathon. I wasn't ready to retire from that distance because it had given me such positive feelings.

⚮

Meanwhile, I first had to get through another Winterman race. The previous year's race had been so tough because of the poor weather conditions; this time I would come better prepared. The night before the race, I laid out my warmest hat that tied under the chin, a wicking hat for underneath it, a neck warmer, a base layer long-sleeved shirt and pants, winter running pants, a T-shirt, a long-sleeved shirt, a vest, my bright green neon waterproof wind jacket (bright so I could be found if I got lost in a snow drift), not one but two pairs of gloves with hot packs inside, wicking socks, wool socks, running shoes and my wonderful crampons that would prevent me from losing my footing. With all that clothing, it just might take more time to get dressed for the race than to run it!

I had a nightmare about the race that night. I dreamed I arrived at the race site totally unequipped for winter, so I had to run laps inside a gymnasium rather than run outdoors with everyone else, and because of that I wasn't given a finisher's medal. I guess I subconsciously suffered from anxiety about the race. I tossed and turned much of the night before the race. I got out of bed at 6 am. I ate a light carb breakfast, and then Allan dropped me off at the race.

Winter of 2009/2010 had the least amount of snowfall in the past 30 years, but of course it started to snow just before the race began. I wore sunglasses even though the sky was gray because they kept the snowflakes out of my eyes.

The first 5 km loop went quite well. I was properly dressed so I wasn't cold. With my crampons attached to my shoes, I wasn't losing my footing. The last time I'd run the Winterman, I was so slow. This time I decided to try to run faster since the weather wasn't bad. The second 5 km loop was harder and took me a few extra minutes. As I saw the end point in the distance, about 500 meters away, I started sprinting. Well, it felt like I was sprinting, I'm not sure. I was definitely giving it my all and I was suddenly finding it hard to breathe. With the blustery wind, my earflaps on my hat flopped up and down as if I were about to take flight. I looked like a cross between Elmer Fudd and the Flying Nun as I crossed the finish line.

❦

One of the books I read that winter was *The Athlete's Way* by world-class endurance athlete Christopher Bergland. I found it to be inspiring and therefore, a useful book to read as the spring half marathon approached. I particularly liked what the author wrote with respect to having won first place in the Triple Iron Man event: "It was the hardest challenge of my life, something I thought I could never do. But I did it. There was some emancipation from self-doubt in achieving that goal" (p. 28).

It seemed ironic that he had "some emancipation from self-doubt" after winning the Triple Iron Man—an extreme event that included a 7.2 mile swim, a 336 mile bike ride, and a 78.6 mile run—without rest or sleep. The first time I ran a half marathon, I looked at it the same way that Christopher Bergland looked at the Triple Iron Man. It was a big challenge, but I was fully committed. Since then, I've looked at each subsequent race as something I knew I could achieve. It still boggles my mind when I think about how much of an impact our thoughts have over our actions. The shift from self-doubt to self-confidence definitely affects our performance.

In October of 2010, I registered for the personal trainer course and began to study the manual. The first chapter was about fundamental concepts of fitness. I read through it many times, using mnemonic devices and other techniques to memorize various key terms. I would read a page several times and repeat the terms in my head. A moment later when trying to list the terms, I couldn't remember more than a few. I never did have a good memory and it had been more than 20 years since I'd written a university exam. How would I retain all of this new information? I took advantage of the accompanying online course that reviewed the material and provided self-assessment questions for each chapter. I also answered the questions in the study guide as I completed each chapter. After a couple of weeks I had completed a few chapters and I realized I was starting to retain much of the pertinent information. It felt good to use my brain and to learn totally new subject matter. If it were easy, what would be the point?

I wondered if I'd be the oldest student in the class. I suspected many of the participants would be in their twenties, but it didn't really matter. I would be attending for my own knowledge and benefit and for my own growth and personal development. This challenge would take me on a new journey.

As I'd anticipated, I was the oldest student in the class of 10. The youngest was 21. Yet, I felt like I fit in. We were all interested in the course and wanted to learn. Some wanted to carve out a career for themselves as personal trainers. One woman was a gym teacher and wanted to enhance her skills. Two women were bored with their current careers and wanted to go in a new direction. The more I learned, the more I started to think that maybe I really did want to train clients. I really wanted to inspire and motivate others to be their best. First, I would have to pass the written theory exam in late November and the second step would be the practical exam which I planned on doing in the winter. Step by step, like a runner in a race, I would get closer to my goal and when I crossed that finish line, I would celebrate all my hard work. Only then would I truly know what I would want to do next.

I wrote the personal trainer certification exam at the end of November. I had studied a couple of hours per day for nearly a month following the completion of the course. As the exam date approached, I became somewhat anxious. My fear of failure intensified. Everyone said I would pass with flying colors but I wasn't so confident. I figured I'd rather be over-prepared than poorly prepared. As it turned out, I was very well-prepared. As I whipped through each of the first 20 or so multiple choice questions, I thought to myself that this exam is just too easy. I wondered if the other examinees found it as easy. When I was a high school student, my Canadian histoire (that's history taught in French) teacher, Madame Silverstein, told my parents at parent-teacher interviews that I was an excellent student but that I wasn't good at multiple choice tests. I think Madame Silverstein unknowingly scarred me for life because I always remembered her remark. It instilled in me a fear of multiple choice tests. Ironically, decades later while working in high tech, I designed and developed multiple choice tests and later managed the development of them for software specialist certification exams.

As I continued to answer the questions on the personal trainer exam with ease, I thought of Madame Silverstein for a fleeting moment. Maybe she was wrong. Maybe I just didn't enjoy Canadian history or the way she taught the class. That was 1980 and here I was 30 years later, performing extremely well on a multiple choice exam.

What had begun as a just-for-fun goal had become a meaningful pursuit, one that motivated me to work harder than I had anticipated and that caused me some stress. But that's me. When I decide to go for something, I like to give it my best effort. Just like losing weight and getting fit, just like taking up running—becoming certified as a personal trainer was something I was willing to work hard at. With the theory exam behind me and the practical exam planned for the new year, I felt like the hardest part was over. I already felt like a winner. I got an A-plus on the exam. I was so excited.

A couple of months later, I did the practical exam. I was assigned a case study and I had to prepare a written workout program for a fictitious client and demonstrate that I could both meet the client's needs and teach the client according to a lengthy checklist of criteria. Again, I prepared myself very well and practiced with my client who was role-played by my friend Paula. The exam went well and the examiner scored me 95 percent. I was so happy. The next day I made the following entry on my Facebook page:

"Passed my final certification exam last night. Now I am a personal fitness trainer. When I retired four years ago at age 42, I was overweight, ate tons of fast food, and rarely did any physical activities. For a year I puttered around the gym. When I turned 44, I decided to make some serious changes. The first thing I changed was my attitude. I truly believe that fitness is mostly mental. I discovered a passion for fitness—a far cry from my past life as a couch potato/desk jockey. After I lost the excess weight and felt fit, I became interested in learning more and wanted to pursue personal fitness trainer certification; but I felt insecure since this was foreign territory compared to my educational background and career history. Well, I applied myself, studied hard, and did well. So, in a way my journey is complete. From couch potato to fitness warrior and trainer…or is my new journey just beginning?"

Fast-forward to winter of 2012. By that time, I had a year of personal training experience under my belt. I'd worked one-on-one with people young and old. I'd helped clients set and work towards their goals. I continued to learn and grow as I researched individual situations. I was training clients with a wide range of common and some not-so-common health issues including overweight, obesity, arthritis, injury-related pain, limited mobility, Parkinson's disease, autism, cardiovascular disease, depression, and low self-esteem. By that time, I'd also taught many types of group fitness classes.

Now I wanted to go beyond the bricks and mortar of the gym. I wanted to reach a larger audience and spread my message about the benefits of a healthy lifestyle. I came up with the idea to reach both fit people and those who most needed encouragement. I'd write a fitness column. But where?

I approached the editor of a local community newspaper with a proposal for a fitness column. I was pleasantly surprised when the editor gave me the green light as well as free reign to write whatever I wanted. With a readership of several thousand people, I now had a much wider audience.

Immediately after my first article was printed, I began to receive positive feedback. It started with a few friends and then I began to get kudos from people at the gym—some of whom I didn't even know. Within a few months, people around town would come up to me and tell me they liked my column or that they were trying to implement some of the tips or exercises I'd written about. I felt like a pseudo-celebrity! More importantly, I felt as though I was making a positive impact by inspiring and educating the masses.

In 2013, I had the opportunity to attend a motivational talk by the famous TV talk show host Oprah Winfrey. One of her themes was about reaching for and working towards your dreams step by step. The very next day, I received an unexpected phone call. One of the moms at Joshua's school was inviting me to give a fitness presentation to her women's group. I was delighted! This was exactly the next step in my personal vision. I just hadn't realized it until I received the phone call. I was training clients, I was writing a fitness column, and next I wanted to deliver motivational talks to groups. Public speaking would be the next platform from which I could inspire others to reach for their dreams.

I delivered an interactive motivational talk to the women's group and a week later I gave a motivational talk at a women's running clinic. I then proposed a motivational workshop to the manager at the community center where I worked. She embraced the idea.

"If you will it, it is no dream." So said Theodore Herzl. It's true.

When you believe something is possible, you can picture it—and that is precisely the moment when you can begin to take action and shape your dream into a reality. I believed I had something to share that could help others and I was finding ways to make it happen. Before I knew it, I'd been invited to deliver a talk at a conference. From there, more engagements would follow.

⁂

I went to my family doctor a couple of weeks before the Ottawa half marathon, complaining of on-again, off-again sore hips that I'd experienced in recent years. I wondered whether running was causing or aggravating the problem. She told me that "people my age shouldn't run" and that our bodies were not designed for long periods of running. She suggested I abandon running and take up swimming. I knew the many benefits of water-based exercise since I'd recently researched that topic and written an article on it.

I booked an appointment with my chiropractor. I've always had confidence in him because of his sports-oriented, common-sense approach. I told him what my family doctor had said. He told me that her way of thinking was "old school" and that if I was happy running, I should stick with it since it has so many health benefits. He attributed my sore hips to my tight hamstrings. After a few Active Release Technique treatments on my hamstrings, and using a foam roller after my workouts as he suggested, my hips felt fine. I decided to follow his advice and keep on running. I'm not saying that my family physician was necessarily wrong with regards to running, but I decided to listen to my chiropractor and to my inner voice. I wasn't ready to give up running.

⁂

I ran my tenth half marathon in May of 2013 at the Ottawa Race Weekend—a huge event that consisted of multiple races and some 44,000 participants. Despite the horrific Boston Marathon bombings that had taken place just a month prior, a whopping 100,000 spectators turned out in support of the runners. I had trained well and I was raring to go.

With unusually cool temperatures, overcast skies, and a fresh

146

breeze—perfect weather conditions for running—I ran a strong race. I managed to keep up with the 2:15 pace bunny for the first 10 kilometers, achieving my best 10K in 63 minutes. Although the pace bunny disappeared into the distance a short time later as I slowed down, I still managed to run well. I was thrilled to finish with a new personal best of 2 hours and 23 minutes.

I think I subconsciously wanted to prove to myself that even though I was now 49 years old, and even though my doctor had suggested I give up running, I still had the ability to enjoy running and to keep getting better at it. Not only did I have my best time ever, but instead of feeling depleted and exhausted after the race, I felt energized.

I believed in myself. I was determined to succeed. I was turning each of my dreams and visions into a reality.

Gloria Schwartz

Personal Best Practices

o   Consider the possibilities.

o   Create a personal vision.

o   Believe in yourself. If you don't, who will?

o   Don't be afraid to take the road less travelled.

o   Ask not "Why?" Ask "Why not?!"

o   Don't empower others to hold you back with labels.

o   Just when it seems like your journey is ending, be prepared for the new one that's about to begin.

o   Take the actions needed to convert your dreams into reality.

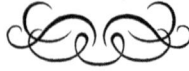

11 REDEMPTION

A moment of visual clarity gives us a glimpse of who we can become.

Poor lifestyle choices and disregard for one's health may provide instant gratification. Unfortunately, more often than not, they also eventually result in the development of chronic or acute medical conditions and a decreased quality of life.

Each of us can find redemption at any point in our lives through faith, belief in oneself, or a combination of the two. God truly does help those who help themselves. What a glorious partnership. Each of us has the free will to make our own choices. Even when we have the knowledge, we don't necessarily make the right choices. Poor choices are not always due to a lack of information, although that can be a contributing factor.

Just as smokers know the negative effects of their habit (it's hard not to know since graphic images of smoking-related diseases are printed on the cigarette packages), people who are inactive and eat poorly do so not necessarily due to a lack of knowledge, but often due to a lack of willpower, commitment, or belief. Trust me, I've been there. We know that a healthy lifestyle can lead to a longer life or a better quality of life. Those facts should be sufficient motivation for each of us to adopt and maintain a more active and healthier lifestyle, but supplying individuals with scientific information about health benefits may not be enough to alter beliefs and behaviors. Sometimes we just don't have all of the tools. We want to feel more energetic, to look better, and to be healthier, yet something holds us back.

We have to be mentally prepared, in the right stage of readiness, to embark on our own individual journey. We have to be in the right frame of mind to stay the course and to develop a passion for fitness. When we have an aha! moment—a moment of visual clarity that defines who we are and gives us a glimpse of who we can become— then our willpower that was dormant within us all along rises to the surface. That is when our inner warrior emerges. It's an awakening. And that's the moment when we can make a lifelong commitment to a fit and healthy lifestyle, and more importantly, to ourselves.

Though we may have lived for many years with poor lifestyle habits—perhaps all of our lives—each day brings with it a new opportunity to be redeemed. It's never too late to start fresh, to take those first few steps in the right direction. We can unlearn old patterns. We can replace negative behaviors with new, positive ones.

We can retrain our brains by thinking in new, more productive ways. Even if we have given up and are focused on illness, we can learn to focus on wellness. We can regain a sense of control over our destinies. Instead of being lackadaisical, we can become enthusiastic. We can learn skills that help us remove or reduce physical and mental barriers that others have imposed on us or that we have imposed on ourselves. We can learn to embrace our true selves rather than sit back and wish we were someone else. By accepting ourselves, we can learn to praise and love ourselves. Loving ourselves is not a permission slip to remain fat, at risk, or unhealthy; rather, it's a golden ticket to a better life. If we're not on the right path, we need to get off of it. Embracing the whole package—even our flaws and foibles—liberates us and makes us feel worthy of change.

Step by step, we can become a better version of ourselves. Life itself is a journey and each of us is a work in progress. The process of change is neither fast nor easy. It may be a long and arduous road. The things that are most important may be the most difficult and require the most attention and effort.

For years, doctors told me I'd soon be on dialysis and there was not much I could do. Few preventative actions were prescribed. I was given a fatalistic prognosis. Only when I finally made up my mind to take control and drop the victim mentality, did I realize that I had the capacity to truly help myself.

For now, my kidney function remains relatively stable. I believe much of this stabilization has been due to my lifestyle changes. This is always the best news possible barring any future medical discoveries that would allow for kidney tissue regeneration, as opposed to the current medical options for kidney failure patients—dialysis or transplantation. Right now there is no pill to cure kidney disease. Unlike the heart, our kidneys are not muscles. We can't strengthen them. The damage that's been done is done. But who knows what science has in store for me or for any of us? As my 90-year-old father tells me, a sudden breakthrough could change all that. He's lived long enough to see countless inventions and discoveries that would have seemed unimaginable in his youth—everything from insulin and heart transplants, to man on the moon, computers, and cell phones. At present, stem cell research holds great promise for curing many diseases. Maybe someday human kidneys will be grown in a lab, making dialysis, dangerously long waits for kidney donations, and anti-rejection drugs that have side effects, things of the past.

These past few years, my nephrologist continues to tell me that my kidneys are pretty stable. After all the ups and down and overly pessimistic "expert" prognoses, I made a decision to just get on with life. Worrying can kill you prematurely! I know people who were healthy as a horse when I was first diagnosed with kidney disease at age 31, and who've since passed away unexpectedly due to accidents or illness. We never know what is in the plan for us, but we can do our best to improve our odds.

I know that for the past several years, I have been doing a lot to take care of myself physically and mentally. There is always room for improvement; however, I am convinced that the changes I've made to my lifestyle have had a positive cumulative effect and that I have been able to have some control over what I once was told was out of my hands. I made choices and I continue to make choices every day. I'm not claiming that I cured myself. That would be unrealistic. What I did is help myself. You can help yourself too, regardless of your situation. By focusing on whole-body health, including mental health, you can strengthen your mind and body even if certain parts are damaged. Instead of focusing on the parts that don't work well and feeling helpless, focus on improving your overall health.

Life is a balancing act for most of us. Eat this and feel happy or deny oneself that pleasure and feel cheated. When we train ourselves to believe that we are not actually cheating ourselves by missing out on a treat, but rather, we are treating ourselves by respecting our bodies and taking care of our health, then the scales shift and it becomes easier to live better. I came to realize that what I am doing is good for me in the big picture and has probably improved my chances of living longer with a better quality of life. I stopped crying over what might happen down the road and realized how fortunate I am today. I came to the point where I could accept my disease as a physical and mental challenge and use it to make myself stronger, rather than allow it to define me. I even embraced my disease as an opportunity to help others. When all of these choices—*my* choices—aligned, I knew that I had found redemption.

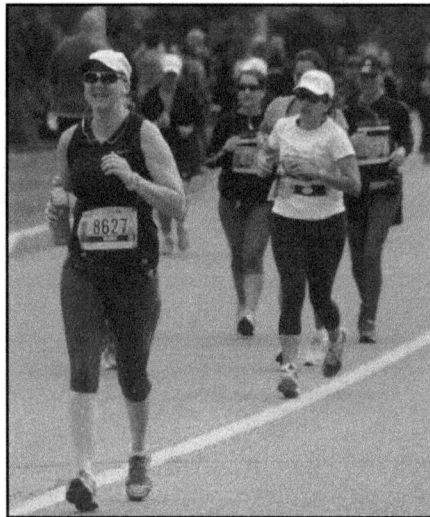

Running my 11th half marathon. This was the last one before I turned 50, but I knew there would be more to come down the road.

Some people go through life with blinders on. They ruminate about their personal problems. They dwell on their medical ailments, no matter how minor. They focus on their shortcomings. They complain about all the negatives they see in themselves and they forget to be grateful for all that they are and all that they have. They dismiss their own potential and all of the possibilities awaiting them if only they were willing to act. They look straight ahead and wonder why the changes they desire seem beyond their reach. They talk and talk about what they want to do but never do it.

At the other end of the spectrum are the people who deny they have problems. Some of them suffer from ailments that they've been diagnosed with, perhaps diabetes, or kidney or heart disease. Others can't function properly day to day because of issues that are aggravated by their excess body weight, such as aching backs, knees, and hips. They may easily get out of breath. Yet, they fool themselves into believing that if they ignore it, the problem will disappear. They make excuses. They lay blame. They ask, "Why me?" They want to feel better, but they're not willing to put in the effort, or they have no idea how to proceed. They are unable to help themselves. They may be afraid to ask for help. They suffer in silence. They do not self-reflect. They do not learn from their mistakes. They do not harness life's lessons. They do not look for opportunities. If there are tools and resources right in front of their noses, they do not see them. I used to be one of those people.

You need to become aware of everything and everyone around you that's an available resource. If only you'd notice, and more importantly, grab onto those opportunities, you could improve the quality of your life.

If you can't see where you came from or what's going on around you, you get stuck. If you don't know where you want to go or you can't envision where you are going, how are you going to get there? Take off your blinders. Introspect. Recognize your shortcomings but appreciate your gloriousness too. Never give up hope! Destiny does, indeed, play a role; but remember that you have the power to intercept and chart your own course. I know you can do it, but it doesn't really matter what I think; you must believe you can do it.

You deserve to become the version of yourself that you dream of. Maybe you already are. Only you can decide. Are you ready and willing to work with your blueprint to map out a fit and healthy future? Whatever journey you choose to embark on, I hope to see you at the finish line. I know that if you want it badly enough, you can achieve your personal best. Until then, I wish you a wonderfully fulfilling adventure, and Godspeed.

Gloria Schwartz

Personal Best Practices

o Accept that which you cannot change. Change that which you cannot accept.

o Stop making excuses.

o Whatever choices you make, push beyond mediocrity. Refuse to accept less than you deserve from yourself and for yourself. Strive to be your personal best.

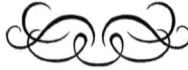

BIBLIOGRAPHY

Allen, James. (2008). *As A Man Thinketh*. New York: Penguin.

Bergland, Christopher. (2007). *The Athlete's Way: Sweat and the Biology of Bliss*. USA: St. Martin's Press.

Dyer, Wayne W. (1989). *You'll See It When You Believe It: The Way to Your Personal Transformation*. New York: HarperCollins Publishers.

Ettinger, Steve. (2008). *Twinkie Deconstructed: My Journey to Discover How the Ingredients Found in Processed Foods are Grown, Mined (Yes, Mined), and Manipulated into What America Eats*. U.S.A.: Plume Paperback.

Izzo, John. (2008). *The Five Secrets You Must Discover Before You Die*. California: Berrett-Koehler Publishers, Inc.

Karnazes, Dean. (2005). *Ultra Marathon Man: Confessions of an All-Night Runner*. New York: Penguin Group.

Murakami, Haruki. (2009). *What I Talk About When I Talk About Running*. Canada: Vintage Canada.

Reno, Tosca. (2006). *The Eat-Clean Diet, Fast Fat-Loss That Lasts Forever*. Canada: Robert Kennedy Publishing.

Sharma, Robin S. (1997). *The Monk Who Sold His Ferrari: A Fable About Fulfilling Your Dreams and Reaching Your Destiny*. Mumbai: Jaico Publishing House.

Zahab, Ray. (2007). *Running for My Life: On the Road with Extreme Runner Ray Zahab*. Canada: Insomniac Press.

CONTACT INFORMATION

To order copies of
Personal Best: Train Your Brain and Transform Your Body for Life, go to:
www.amazon.com

For news and tips, go to:
www.facebook.com/personalbestthebook

To book Gloria Schwartz for a speaking engagement, email:
info@personalbestthebook.com

www.ingramcontent.com/pod-product-compliance
Lightning Source LLC
Chambersburg PA
CBHW050125280326
41933CB00010B/1252